# THE SOCIAL CONSEQUENCES OF FACIAL DISFIGUREMENT

# The Social Consequences of Facial Disfigurement

MICHAEL J. HUGHES

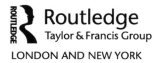

Routledge
Taylor & Francis Group

LONDON AND NEW YORK

First published 1998 by Ashgate Publishing

Reissued 2018 by Routledge
2 Park Square, Milton Park, Abingdon, Oxon, OX14 4RN
711 Third Avenue, New York, NY 10017, USA

*Routledge is an imprint of the Taylor & Francis Group, an informa business*

Publisher's Note
The publisher has gone to great lengths to ensure the quality of this reprint but points out that some imperfections in the original copies may be apparent.

Disclaimer
The publisher has made every effort to trace copyright holders and welcomes correspondence from those they have been unable to contact.

A Library of Congress record exists under LC control number: 97077383

ISBN 13: 978-1-138-36018-1 (hbk)
ISBN 13: 978-0-429-43326-9 (ebk)

# Contents

# List of tables

# Introduction

People who are facially disfigured are often considered not quite whole, not quite normal, or not quite acceptable. How do they experience reactions to their disfigurement? Do they feel disadvantaged? If so, how do they compensate? How do professional people such as doctors, nurses and social workers try to help them? How could that help be improved?

These are the basic questions underlying the present study. The face is important in the formation and maintenance of human relationships. This is illustrated by the many verbal expressions involving the word 'face' which occur in everyday language - 'losing face', 'facing up to it', 'two-faced', and 'about face', for example. Literature too abounds with references to the face; the Penguin Dictionary of Quotations lists 64 well-known citations, from the cataclysmic consequences of 'the face that launched a thousand ships' to the private anguish of Blake when speaking to his patron Thomas Butts about his own distinctive appearance:

O! why was I born with a different face?
Why was I not born like the rest of my race?

The face is exposed, unlike many other parts of the body, and constitutes our preliminary mode of recognition of people. Encounters with strangers rely heavily on the impact of initial appearance. There are many studies which show that unsatisfactory first impressions will prevent people from attempting to pursue an acquaintance. Consequently, anyone who is facially impaired, either in appearance or in damage to sensory organs, is at a serious social disadvantage. Even if the audio-visual system is undamaged, facial impairment alone can inhibit communication, since much communication relies on non-verbal cues supplied by facial expression.

The effect of disfigurement may also be severe in encounters with known others, if the range of non-verbal aids to complete communication is restricted. Facial disfigurement may be accompanied by oral disfigurement, which may impede eating; given the significance of eating as a social activity, the person who feels unable or too self-conscious to eat with others sustains a further isolation.

## Aims of the study

This study was established with the following aims:

1. To describe the nature of facial disfigurement, and the characteristics of those who are disfigured;

2. To describe the causes of disfigurement and deformity;

3. To investigate the social consequences of facial disfigurement;

4. To understand the means which people adopt to overcome the difficulties posed by disfigurement - people who are disfigured, and those who endeavour to help them;

5. To describe the physical, social and psychological consequences of professional intervention;

6. To discover what further can be done by professionals to mitigate the effects of disfigurement and deformity.

## Origin of the study

My interest in the subject first began when I was principal social worker at the Royal Victoria Infirmary in Newcastle upon Tyne. The chief maxillo-facial technician at the hospital, the person responsible for making artificial parts of the body - from false teeth to false ears - raised the issue of emotional support for people whose face had been mutilated by illness or trauma. Previously I had assumed that his role was restricted to the sculpting of acceptable replacement parts for the body, but he was able to show in many instances that those for whom he worked had no other form of human support; they were very isolated people, and he was sometimes the only source of encouragement for those whose clinical needs had abated and who required much less attention from surgical staff than previously. I met some of the people with whom and for whom he worked, and was impressed by the extent of their physical mutilation, but more than that by their strong need for support and encouragement - an elderly man whose face had been eroded by a progressive malignancy, a young man whose ear had been lost in a fight, an elderly woman whose nose had been removed because of cancer - they presented cogent evidence that here were hidden personal needs and difficulties; they were hidden because in every instance a withdrawal from social interaction was described, and on the whole these needs were not being met satisfactorily.

This then was the beginning of my interest and concern, which have instigated and motivated this research.


## Language

Two aspects of language need to be mentioned here. The first is the use of the words 'disfigured' and 'deformed'. Although the social consequences of disfigurement and deformity may in a general sense be similar, the two concepts are distinct, and throughout this work will be used in a precise and consistent way.

Deformity refers to a condition which is in some sense congenital; the condition, or predisposition to the condition, will have been acquired by the time of birth. This may simply be a slightly unusual feature, such as a large nose, or ears which stick out; it may be a severe congenital syndrome of physical characteristics, such as Apert's syndrome, or it may be a syndrome which has amongst other things some physical attributes, such as Down's syndrome. Some may find the expression 'deformity' unacceptable, since they feel that it stigmatises the individual. No such stigma is intended by the term, which literally does refer to a variation from the appearance of the majority. Any stigma associated with the term arises from its inappropriate use as a means of excluding or ridiculing people.

Disfigurement, on the other hand, refers to a condition which has been acquired since birth, through some means other than congenital.

This is likely to be, broadly, through a physical trauma or through illness. Trauma will include injury through burns, cuts and mutilation (through fights or road traffic accidents, for example). The principal illness which occasions facial disfigurement is cancer, and much of this study, particularly the field study, concentrates on this source of disfigurement.

The title of the thesis refers only to disfigurement, but issues concerning congenital deformity are also addressed, particularly in the review of literature.

The second point which must be considered and explained at this point is the expression 'plastic surgery'. This does not refer to the materials used, but rather to the earlier meaning of the word plastic, used to describe a process of moulding and shaping. This is exactly what is required in the modifying and rebuilding of the face, and plastic surgeons are also concerned with the shaping of other parts of the body. Reconstructive surgery is one element of this. A further element is cosmetic surgery, which refers to intention as much as technique; it is used to denote facial modification where previously there had been no serious abnormality, as in the case of those who wish to eliminate the signs of ageing, or those who aspire to perfect appearance, or those who wish to remove fatty tissue.

**Types of disfigurement**

It has already been suggested that abnormalities of the face are occasioned by either an illness or trauma, or were present at birth. The latter are more accurately known as deformity. The following list, while not exhaustive, amplifies this typology, by describing some of the principal causes of facial disfigurement and deformity:

1.  Congenital syndromes - these are numerous. Some possess symptoms which are exclusively ones of physical appearance. Others happen to include such symptoms amongst others, for example Down's syndrome. The child or young person with Down's syndrome will have a range of concerns, including moderate to severe learning difficulties, but they will always include a characteristic facial and oral appearance. Many children and young adults with congenital syndromes are helped considerably by reconstructive surgery; this may be called for partly to minimise the different appearance, and partly to aid physical functioning - breathing, eating, sleeping. Reconstructive work has been carried out on children with Down's syndrome, although this has caused some controversy, as some feel that the balance of effort should be put into convincing society that children whose appearance, behaviour or ability is different from most should be absorbed and

accepted into that society.

2.    Lesser congenital deformities and deformity occasioned by birth trauma. The most common instance of this is the cleft lip and palate. This too is helped substantially by surgery, both in infancy and subsequently, and often the residual deformity is restricted to mild scarring.

3.    Facial attributes which are ethnic characteristics. These are not necessarily deformities, but may be seen as such by some people, especially when they feel unsure or insecure about their inclusion in their own or a new cultural setting. Such people frequently make use of reconstructive surgery, in order to merge more into what they see as the acceptable group - Jewish people who wish to reduce their noses in order to look American, or Chinese people who wish to eradicate the characteristic angle of their eyes.

4.    Other facial characteristics which are also not intrinsically deformities, but may be seen as such by the self-conscious person - for example the child who is teased because his ears stick out. Reconstructive surgery may be of assistance here, provided that the expectations of the results are realistic.

5.    Burns - these are most painful injuries, and so is their treatment, which is principally through one or more processes of grafting skin taken from elsewhere on the body. The results are rarely perfect, and scarring of the site from which skin is taken - the donor site - may also be an issue.

6.    Disfigurement through accident - cuts and scars resulting from car accidents, mutilation through fighting (such as the young man described above whose ear was bitten off in a fight). Results of surgery to address these injuries are often good, since the individual may be otherwise healthy, and the blood supply is strong.

7.    Disfigurement through cancer - this represents a major theme of this study, and the field study is focused on the subject. Cancer which presents in the head and neck may require surgery in order to excise the malignant cells. This may leave a cavity or deficit, and will frequently leave scarring. It is

important to note that on many occasions it is not the cancer itself which is mutilating, but the surgery which is designed to cure it. In many instances it is both.

Oral cancer is the sixth most common malignancy in the United Kingdom; in men it is the fourth most common. Its incidence (1980 figures) is at the rate of 1.3 per thousand in urban areas, and 0.9 per thousand in rural areas.

8.    There is a small amount of disfigurement which is genuinely caused by surgeons. The most common form of this is the carrying out of facial operations by those who are not skilled to do so, or who have undertaken a procedure ill-advisedly. In the course of my study I met a small number of people who came to the surgeons with whom I was working in an attempt to have the results of the earlier surgery minimised.

**Surgical responses**

To most of the situations described above virtually the only possible clinical response is surgery. The exception is cancer, where a number of options are present. For skin cancer present on the face, removal by laser beam has been successful in recent years. For head and neck cancer, the most probable alternative to surgery is radiotherapy, the use of radioactivity to destroy malignant cells. In many instances either surgery or radiotherapy may be used, and patients may then be asked to express a preference.

Since the Second World War, when Sir Archibald McIndoe conducted his pioneering work at the Queen Elizabeth Hospital, East Grinstead, rapid progress has been made in the development of materials and techniques used in plastic surgery. The materials which have been developed have assisted the skills of the surgeon, for example steel, titanium and silicon.

However, it is the use of natural materials which has contributed most to developments: in other words, the use of a vast range of parts of the body to restore the contour of the face - pelvic bone to make good the space in the jaw, abdominal tissue to replace the excised cheek, skin split or stretched to make it go further, even the tissue from the buttocks to replace the tissue on the nose.

Along with the advances in the actual materials, there have been major developments in the techniques used to get the most out of these materials. The most important of these has been micro-vascular surgery.

When tissue is moved from one part of the body to another, it is important that a blood supply is established at the new site for the transplanted material. For many years, this was achieved by leaving the donor material attached to the original site, as well as to the new site, until it was certain that a supply was being provided by the host site. This might take several weeks. The tissue could then be detached in a further operation from its original position, and trimmed to fit the new position more precisely.

One aspect of this procedure was that more tissue was 'raised' from the donor site than was ultimately necessary, since it would need to stretch from the donor area to the host area. The stretched piece of skin and tissue is known as a pedicle. In order to prevent the pedicle from deteriorating during the waiting period, its open sides were curved round and fastened together, thus making what is known as a tubed pedicle.

By means of a tubed pedicle, skin, muscle, and even bone, may be moved around the body, for example from the shoulder to the face, or from the wrist to the face. However, the process is restricted by only being suitable for moving tissue from an area near the head - the shoulder, chest, or upper arm, for example, and also the forearm, which can be moved and held in position near the face. However, it is also possible to carry out a two stage transfer, by attaching the required tissue from elsewhere (for example the thigh) to the wrist; when blood flow has been established there, the original site can be detached, and the process repeated from wrist to face. When I visited the Mayo Clinic, I spoke to a young woman who had a congenital deformity involving the absence of one eye and orbit or socket. An orbit was created for her, using the wrist as the workbench, with tissue from elsewhere. When the socket was ready, a grafting operation was carried out moving the newly-grown orbit from the wrist to its proper place.

All of this is most elaborate, involving patients and staff in two and three stage procedures. In Marjorie Jackson's book *The Boy David*, there are photographs of David at various stages of the grafting process. They illustrate the laborious, painful and time-consuming nature of the process, as well as the interim unsightliness of the newly-grafted tubed pedicles.

More recently, techniques have been developed which eliminate much of this many-staged procedure. These have been made possible through micro-surgery - the use of microscopes in the operating theatre in order to carry out much more refined and precise procedures. The most important of these is micro-vascular surgery, the linking of blood vessels to each other.

Consequently, when a piece of tissue is moved, it can take with it its own supply system; the blood vessels which supply it are taken too, and sewn to blood vessels in the new area. Thus blood supply is established in only one process, making it possible to carry out a many-staged procedure in one day - removal of malignant tissue, the raising of donor material from elsewhere, attaching it to the new site, establishing blood supply, and trimming the tissue to achieve a satisfactory appearance. Sometimes a further minor procedure is required to complete this trimming.

An illustration of this procedure is provided in the next section.


**The surgical process**

Early in my study, I was invited to visit the Department of Plastic and Reconstructive Surgery at St. James' Hospital, Leeds, by Mr. Andrew Batchelor, consultant plastic surgeon.

Mr. Batchelor had expressed interest in the study, and felt that a useful preliminary to my involvement would be the observation of a major operation.

I therefore spent the whole day in theatre, observing an operation which lasted from 8.30 a.m. until 4.30 p.m. The purpose of the operation was to transplant bone from the pelvis of the patient to his cheek, to replace the bone which had been removed because of the presence of malignant cells.

At the time of the removal of the carcinoma, the area was covered by a flap of soft tissue taken from elsewhere in the body. This had proved insufficient to restore the contour of the face, and the patient complained of dribbling, because of the absence of supporting bone.

The advances described in the previous section are only very recent, and had the technique been available originally, Mr. Batchelor would have removed the malignant tissue and carried out the bone graft all in one procedure. Now, he had to perform the double operation of opening a donor site, and reopening the host site. The patient was a man in his fifties, highly motivated to undergo the restoration.

The process was successful, with two qualifications. The bone was excised and resited, and the surgical work was completed adequately, but the feeling of overall success was marred, first by the discovery of a node in the neck, which might be found on analysis to be metastatic, and secondly by the fact that there was still a recess in the patient's cheek. This could have been corrected by the transfer of soft tissue from another donor site, but it was decided to await the outcome of the biopsy, and conduct a further operation if the health of the patient was stable. This decision was taken very rapidly, but with the utmost care. The need to provide the patient with as long and as comfortable a life as possible was paramount. His own likely preference was weighed up, and it was considered that the effect of recovering and finding that not only had the work been stopped but also a secondary cancerous site had been found would have been too distressing. If in addition the new growth proved not to be malignant, the energies of the patient would have been exhausted with no return. It was decided that it was worthwhile to proceed with the original plan, but to go no further. In this way, something would have been achieved for the patient, without subjecting him to unnecessary discomfort.

The sewing of the artery and vein attached to the bone to their host site was fascinating. This phase took some three hours, and was carried out using a surgical microscope.

At the end of the procedure, the main concern of the surgeon, following eight hours of concentrated physical, emotional and mental exertion, was that he should telephone the patient's wife as soon as possible, to tell her that her husband was now recovering well from a long and very serious, but quite successful, operation.


**The present study**

Several components contribute to the fulfilment of the aims of the study which were outlined at the beginning of the introduction. First of all, in Part I, the literature review, the origins of disfigurement and deformity are examined from a range of perspectives, together with societal responses to it, and responses of disfigured people themselves. The achievements of professionals in correcting disfigurement and deformity are considered, and the outcomes of professional involvement are evaluated, particularly as they have affected the functioning of disfigured people.

The literature falls naturally into four parts. Chapter One takes a sociological approach, examining in particular the work of Erving Goffman in relation to stigma. With the exception of Kai Erikson's contribution, the remaining sociological thought referred to has derived from Goffman.

In Chapter Two, the unique contribution of Frances Macgregor is described and evaluated. Frances Macgregor began her academic work as a social anthropologist, and applied this approach to the study of facial deformity. Her career and writing extends over forty years, and has had a major impact on clinical practice in the United States.

Chapter Three draws together a number of contributions from professionals, principally surgeons and psychologists. These contributions do not form one coherent whole, and frequently the writers make little reference to one another, suggesting that our knowledge of the subject has not been advanced as systematically as it should have been.

Chapter Four is concerned with of the writings of those who are or have been disfigured. All three authors cited (James Partridge, Simon Weston and Christine Piff) were disfigured in adult life, and so are able to describe in detail the process of becoming disfigured, the feelings engendered, and the responses which they made. All of them have views on professional practice, what its value was to them, and in some instances how it could be improved.

Part II contains a description of responses to the needs of disfigured people. One way in which some disfigured people make sense of their situation, and make it bearable, is to group together with others with a similar condition, in order to give and receive advice and support. There are now in existence several mutual help groups for people with a disfigurement or deformity, and their special contribution is evaluated in Chapter Five.

Part III is a report of an empirical study. On the basis of the understanding of disfigurement and deformity derived from the literature study, a series of hypotheses was established which were then tested in a field study. The principal component of this field study was a set of interviews with disfigured people, carried out in order to learn from their experience of becoming disfigured and of adjustment to their new state. The focus of this study, and the reasons for adopting this focus, are described in Chapter Six. The study considers only a sample of people who have undergone surgery for the removal of facial cancer; this is both valuable and limiting -valuable because it considers in depth one very distinct group of people, and limiting because of its exclusion of other important groups, particularly those with congenital deformities.

The study was carried out in two stages: Chapter Seven describes the results of interviews with patients carried out very soon after treatment. Not all of the original 71 patients survived, and so the group seen at second interview was smaller than the original sample. The social characteristics of the survivors are summarised in Chapter Eight. Chapter Nine follows up the same people a year later, in order to examine how far they have settled their lives after the upheaval of illness and treatment. In the final chapter in Part III, Chapter Ten the original hypotheses are reviewed, in order to see whether they have been upheld.

In the Conclusion, the threads of the whole study are drawn together by highlighting issues of particular importance, and by suggesting ways in which professionals, particularly social workers, may give help and support to reduce the social and psychological impact of disfigurement.

# PART I
# SPOILED IDENTITY

# 1 The sociology of stigma

Deviance theory has greatly assisted our understanding of the problems of cranio-facial disfigurement and deformity. This body of theory, which was developed in the United States in the early 1960s, seeks to understand societal responses to people who do not fit the stereotypes of the 'normal'. It was originally concerned with deviant behaviour among young people at odds with society - with the drop-outs, with marijuana smoking and petty theft - the complex reactions of a generation which resisted a 'straight' society committed to property ownership and the development of nuclear warheads. Becker's *The Other Side* (1964) [1] was a powerful plea by a group of sociologists for greater tolerance of the unconventional. Edwin Schur's *Victimless Crimes* (1965) [2] with its plea of 'Leave the kids alone' argued that young people were criminalised by the law rather than by their own acts. Deviant appearance was involved in these analyses because deviant young people tended to cultivate a style of dress and presentation which marked them out from the rest of society.

Consideration was extended to the problems of other groups who did not fit the image of the 'normal', such as adult criminals, vagrants, homosexuals, unmarried mothers, mentally ill and mentally and physically handicapped people. The central theme was that deviance existed only in the eye of the beholder: that the stigmatisation of the people who were 'different' was pathological, a means of social control. Thomas Szasz [3] described the origin of 'scapegoating' - the Jewish ritual by which a goat was driven into the wilderness bearing the sins of the people.

## The general theory of deviance

In this new literature, and in much which followed, no clear distinction was made between problems of behaviour and problems of appearance:

15

the concepts of 'scapegoating' and 'stigma' carried the assumption that the deviant was identifiable - and conversely that deviant appearance could be regarded as a predictor of deviant behaviour.

Perhaps the clearest account of the general theory of deviance is that presented by Kai Erikson.[4] This challenges the convention that deviant behaviour is a threat to a society, and that norms and controls are established in order to protect the society from harm. On the contrary, he argues, deviance is needed by society in order to mark the boundary between acceptable and unacceptable behaviour.

Members of the society decide what space they occupy collectively within the boundaries. They know where the group begins and ends, and what it feels like to belong to the group. A useful way, or perhaps the only way, to mark the boundaries is to note how the members behave and perhaps the best boundary marker is deviant behaviour, since it represents 'the most extreme variety of conduct to be found within the experience of the group.' So, when deviant persons and agencies of control have dealings with each other, these are boundary marking mechanisms. They tell us where the norm is, and how much variation and diversity the norm can tolerate, 'before it begins to lose its distinct structure, its cultural integrity.' So, far from being disruptive impingements on a society, they are an integral part of it:

> Thus deviance cannot be dismissed simply as behaviour which disrupts stability in society, but may itself be, in controlled quantities, an important condition for preserving stability. [5]

In support of this principal statement, Erikson describes the following characteristics of deviant behaviour:

> Many of the features which cause the judgement to be made about the individual are external to the act or characteristic under consideration, for example, social class, past record of offending, how much sorrow or contrition he shows for his act, cleanliness, tidiness, and articulacy. So some people carrying out certain activities are labelled deviant whereas others who carry out the same act are not. So, how does the community decide what is deviant and what is not? Conventional wisdom is that society sets up controls to protect itself from harm. But in fact it is not necessarily the case that things that they decide are deviant are harmful to society, and here Erikson draws on the experience of anthropology to illustrate the point.

Perhaps the most interesting problem for those of us who lean over into the applied areas of the field, however, is to ask whether we have anything to learn from those cultures which permit re-entry into normal social life for persons who have spent a period of time in the deviant ranks and no longer have any special need to remain there.[6]

A norm is not found expressed as a single rule. Rather it is the sum of the ties the community has stated what it feels about a particular issue. So it has a history, and eventually it takes on sufficient status to become a precedent. Every time the society declares an act deviant, it is a re-statement of the norm.

Deviant behaviour is usually only a very small part of the behaviour of the individual. Most of the time he or she may be conforming, but it is the deviant element which draws the label to him or her.

The community has taken note of a few scattered particles of behaviour and has decided that they reflect what kind of person he 'really' is.[7]

The decision to label somebody deviant has three stages - confrontation, judgement and placement. They are usually public acts, with a fairly flamboyant, dramatic flavour to them - for example, the criminal trial. However, the reversal into the centre of society is scarcely ever as public, for example, the quiet discharge from prison of the prisoner, or the release of the patient from psychiatric hospital.

In summary, deviance is not a breaking of the boundaries of the social structure, or a failure of the system, but rather a means of marking the outer restrictions or boundaries of the system, a positive, useful force. This is not to say that the system causes the crises, but it makes use of them to the best advantage of the community or society.


## Deviance theory applied to appearance

Erikson's theory of deviance helps explain society's approach to the question of appearance. Appearance is a determinant of the acceptability of the person, and society marks the boundary between acceptable and unacceptable appearance, as it does behaviour. There is a range of appearance, as with behaviour, which may be described as 'normal' by a group or by society. In order to confirm the normality of the group, other forms of appearance are judged plain or ugly, which are threats to the accepted norm. Those who do not come within the scope of normal appearance are excluded, but they fulfil a necessary role in relation to those who are viewed as normal.

Appearance may be used to confirm either a group within a society, or the society itself. Young people adopt forms of dress and facial appearance to confirm their normality within the group, and to mark their differentness from the remainder of society, and from older people in particular. The broader society also has conventions about what is acceptable, often related to ethnic characteristics and features. Frances Macgregor's study of those who came for plastic surgery in New York for reduction of their noses revealed that in that society, many people of Jewish or eastern European origin sought to assume the appearance of an Irish person.[8] This is remarkable in view of the superior status of those of Anglo-Saxon origin, but the emphasis was most definitely on 'Irish'.

Within an ethnic group, conventions are held as to what is normal, and this may become more critical when the risks of being abnormal are greater. In a paper delivered to the British Association of Oral and Maxillo-facial Surgeons autumn meeting of 1989, J.F. Yeo of the National University Hospital, Singapore, described the pressures on Asians of Chinese origin who have the congenital feature of a prominent jaw (prognathism) to undergo surgery to have the jaw reduced. The condition is more common in that group than in the European population, but it is still socially unacceptable, and many young people seek surgery (which is usually very successful) to enable them to be accepted and lead a more rewarding social life.

In the United Kingdom, plastic surgeons frequently have discussions with patients and the parents of younger patients about what constitutes deformity. Children attend for the modification of ears which stick out, in order to stop being ridiculed at school. The discussions on whether or not to proceed with surgery are boundary-marking discussions. The fact that they take place illustrates the fact that the matter of what is normal or acceptable is not clear-cut; there is no fixed definition of acceptability. However, no one wishes to be a member of the out-group, and so reassurances by the surgeon that minor differences are within the normal range are often not enough to convince the intending patient.

The degree of deviation from normal appearance is not the sole determinant of acceptance. What is unacceptable in a particular society for one sub-group or in one situation may be acceptable in another. In the present study, elderly, working-class men on more than one occasion dismissed the significance of their disfigurement, saying that 'it would have been different if I were a young lass, or a young lad courting, but at my age who cares?' Appearance is one of a range of indicators which determine whether we should accept someone - others include age, gender, social class, job (high profile or behind the scenes), and temperament.

Consequently, acceptable appearance is hard to define. In addition, the individual carries with him or her a whole unique history of impressions about appearance; the level of tolerance and acceptance of others will vary from person to person, but the collective perceptions and judgements of the majority are a statement of the norm.

The individual is made up of many more components than appearance alone, but appearance is the primary determinant of whether a stranger will look further and get to know the individual.[9] Appearance provides the auspices for making more profound acquaintance. If appearance suggests that a person is not normal, the other may proceed no further in getting to know him or her, in just the same way as small parts of a person's overall behaviour give opportunities for society to decide 'what kind of person he "really" is.'

The labelling of someone as abnormal because of appearance alone is not so formalised as the process which attaches to behaviour. There is no public trial, no formalised committal. However, public declarations do exist of stereotypes of acceptable behaviour - beauty shows, art and photography all present a stylised image of what is normal. Advertising uses our need or urge to stay within this norm by conforming to the purchasing practice of those who look normal. A courageous deviation from this approach was recently taken by Mothercare, who at the instigation of Jimmy Saville used a child with Down's syndrome as one of their models for their 1990 catalogue.

Generally, however, the person who does not match the societal norm of appearance is virtually powerless to move from his or her allotted role and overthrow the negative judgement of others, because appearance is virtually a constant, and far more difficult to alter or disguise than unacceptable behaviour.

In a very real sense, therefore, the disfigured individual is ascribed the deviant role, and is excluded from acceptance by society. He or she lacks the basic currency required to belong to the group, in this case normal appearance, and has little chance of ever resuming a fully accepted place within the community.


## Goffman and stigma

Erving Goffman's *Stigma*[10] extends Erikson's concepts and his own previous work in *Asylums*[11] to a consideration of the mechanisms of stigma and 'spoiled identity'. It is a most important contribution to understanding the issues and difficulties which are presented to those with facial disfigurement, and to understanding the ways in which they and those around them respond. *Stigma* was published in 1963, but there is evidence that Goffman was developing the concepts of stigma and deviance as early as 1957.[12] The subtitle, 'Notes on the Management of Spoiled Identity,' is well-deserved, for this is a most condensed work, filled with headings, definitions and constructs. Many of the concepts are drawn from the work of others, but where these are lacking Goffman describes and names them himself at a rapid rate, and uses them as the raw material from which to build the larger construct. One cannot dip into this work -Goffman assumes one's understanding of earlier definitions throughout the rest of the pages; failure to absorb one page reduces understanding of the next, as each contributes to a well-integrated whole.

Goffman defines stigma as 'something unusual and bad about the moral status of the signifier'.[13] This indeed is the principal sense in which he uses the expression, but he also offers a three-point typology of stigma, which does not match this definition in all respects.

His typology of stigma is three-fold: it can be a physical deformity, and this is the sense in which the Greeks coined the expression. (One early specialist use of the plural of the word in this sense, stigmata, is to denote the marks of the Crucifixion. Subsequently, men and women who possessed this physical attribute were also accorded the attribute of sanctity.) It can refer to a character trait, such as dishonesty, inferred from a behavioural record, such as imprisonment or addiction. It can also refer to the distinctiveness of a tribe, a race or a religion. In the latter case, the stigmatised group or individual are sometimes unrepentant about their stigma -they know that they are stigmatised, but wish to retain the characteristics which endow the stigma -for example, orthodox Jews.

Such a typology is not necessarily helpful for this study. The most important point to note is that stigma may be physical on the one hand, or behavioural and moral on the other. Much of Goffman's analysis is concerned with behaviour rather than with stigma in its original sense. The original sense has the greater bearing on the present study.

It comes about because society categorises people, and assigns to them attributes which are held to be appropriate to that category; each person possesses a social identity - a series of attributes which assist others to categorise them. Social identity may be virtual or actual - virtual social identity is how we think someone should be classified, and actual social identity reflects more accurately his or her attributes if we knew him or her better. Some of these attributes will be discrediting, and Goffman calls such attributes stigmata - undesired differentness from those regarded as 'normals'. The implication is that the stigmatised person is not quite human, unaccepted by themselves and others.

Within such discrediting attributes, Goffman distinguishes between those which are already known to a wide audience, and those which would be damaging if they were so. Those who possess attributes which are already known are 'discredited', while those whose discrediting attributes are not yet known are 'discreditable'.

So, within the first few pages, Goffman has produced a series of carefully defined terms - social identity, virtual and actual, discrediting, discreditable, discredited, normals, and of course stigma itself.

## Strategies to reduce stigma

A range of strategies can be used to reduce the effect of being stigmatised; these are: removal, countering, fighting, avoiding, passing and covering.

Firstly, one can attempt to remove the stigma - in the case of disfigurement this could be attempted through surgery. This in turn may produce the status of someone who used to carry the stigma - a new form of stigma, 'a recovered ...'

Secondly, the person may aim to counter the stigma by acquiring skills not normally seen to be within the grasp of the person with the stigma -for example, sporting activities for those with physical disability, music or swimming for those with a mental handicap.

Next, the individual may fight the stigma:

> ... the person with a shameful differentness can break with what is called reality, and obstinately attempt to employ an unconventional interpretation of the character of his social identity.[14]

The stigmatised person will spend much time and effort in considering the social contacts which he or she is likely to encounter with non-stigmatised people, and to arrange life around avoiding them. This will consume much of their energy:

> Presumably this will have larger consequences for the stigmatised, since more arranging will usually be necessary on

their part.[15]

## 'Passing' and 'covering'

The two strategies which are dealt with in most detail by Goffman are 'passing' and 'covering'. 'Passing' refers to the process of presenting as 'normal', by not disclosing the stigma. People with whom the stigmatised person deals may be divided into the knowing and the unknowing - some may know details about a person's identity, others may not; the stigmatised person lives in a state of uncertainty, as he or she may not be sure who knows and who does not know. The occasions most difficult to manage are not those where there is little likelihood of disclosure, or every appearance of stigma, but rather the broad range in the middle, where people need to conceal from some and expose to others:

> Nearly all matters which are secret are still known to someone, and hence cast a shadow.[16]

The problems which people may wish to conceal in order to pass as normal are ones which most people face at some time, and many will conceal them:

> Because of the great rewards in being considered normal, almost all persons who are in a position to pass will do so on some occasion by intent.[17]

Also, on occasions, it is not proper, or presumes too much on casual acquaintance, to disclose a stigma. Stigmatised individuals

> ...are forced to present themselves falsely in almost all situations, having to conceal their unconventional secrets because of everyone's having to conceal the conventional ones.[18]

'Passing' may be unintended, or totally deliberate. If a person's attempts at passing are later found to be based on features incompatible with others' biographical record of him or her, he or she becomes discredited. So, personal identification may have an impact on social identity (as with the Al Fayid brothers in the Harrods take-over row of 1990. The brothers had previously claimed that they were of aristocratic origin, and when it was disclosed that they were of humbler but perfectly respectable middle class background, the fact that they had lied arguably did them more harm than if they had been open about their origins in the first place ).

The person who passes may find himself or herself at risk of disclosure and discreditation unexpectedly, and must deal with it. In these circumstances the discreditable person learns what people think about his or her particular disadvantage. It is made more difficult if he or she is not sure who knows about the secret:

> What are unthinking routines for normals can become management problems for the discreditable. These problems cannot always be handled by past experience, since new contingencies always arise, making former concealing devices inadequate.[19]

Several techniques are used in order to pass: some conceal the signs of stigma, others present the signs as if they belong to a less discrediting stigma, while others draw a small group into collusive awareness, sometimes using close ones such as family to assist in the concealment.

The individual may also disclose to a larger group, thereby changing voluntarily from discreditable to discredited, and instead manage the difficult social situation which this creates. This process is known as covering, managing the differentness between being discreditable and discredited, and also the difference between mere visibility and positive obtrusiveness. The person makes an evident stigma seem of less consequence. The means of doing so are similar to the techniques used in passing:

> The intent behind such devices such as change in name and change in nose shape is not solely to pass, but also to restrict the way in which a known-about attribute obtrudes itself into the centre of attention, for obtrusiveness increases the difficulty of obtaining easeful inattention regarding the stigma.[20]

As with passing, individuals will organise social situations in order to cover.

When indeed the two do confront each other, stigmatised and non-stigmatised, neither knows how to proceed - how will the stigmatised person be categorised? Will the categorisation be positive or negative? In making an appraisal, the person without stigma will tend not to apply the usual standards and instruments. He or she will self-consciously make allowances for the stigma, viewing minor accomplishments as major, and ascribing all faults to the stigma. For example, if a person is violent or angry, this may be viewed as a re-emergence of a previous mental illness.

When stigmatised people are in public, they are likely to be made to feel that their privacy can more legitimately be invaded than other people's: they can be stared at, or interrogated; their differentness singles them out:

> The implication of these overtures is that the stigmatised individual is a person who can be approached by strangers at will, providing only that they are sympathetic to the plight of persons of his kind.[21]

Stigmatised persons lose their privacy, and non-stigmatised people do not keep the same respectful distance that they would normally maintain.

In order to defend against this invasion, the stigmatised individual will be anxious. So, both stigmatised person and other are most likely to have problems in relating to each other:

> In consequence, attention is furtively withdrawn from its obligatory targets, and self-consciousness and 'other-consciousness' occur, expressed in the pathology of interaction-uneasiness.[22]

## Breaking through

Goffman challenges the commonly accepted view that with greater familiarity and interaction also comes greater acceptance. He first cites several examples of situations in which greater tolerance does follow familiarity.[23] This is the phenomenon described by Davis[24] as 'breaking through' - where for the person whose disadvantage is visible, every new encounter must be explored for its potential for further development, in a most self-conscious manner - Partridge's 'loss of automatic right to acceptance'.[25] Goffman cites the husband-wife relationship as a situation where longer association produces fixed expectations. This is where the argument becomes thin: he does not demonstrate that the husband-wife relationship is essentially stigmatising, although he allows himself a moral outburst suggesting that the wife is degraded:

> Surely it is scandalous.... [26]

Sociological argument ceases when he resorts to

> There are sure to be cases where ...[27]

Perhaps he sees a need to shore up thin argument with exhortation and words of affirmation or reinforcement.


## The own and the wise

Two groups of people will be particularly sympathetic to the stigmatised individual, those whom Goffman calls the Own and the Wise.

The Own are those who share the stigma, and can therefore help the individual to get by, provide moral support, and make him or her feel normal. If the person does use the Own to form his or her frame of reference, as a basis for life organisation, they 'resign [themselves] to a half-world to do so.' This world will be composed of stigmatised individuals like themselves. The individual may find it either painful or boring - having a stigmatising condition means that you have to listen to the stories of others who have the same condition; this may be a comfort to some but to others it may reinforce their differentness from the rest of society.

As part of this process of comfort, many stigmatised people band together into a club or group of those in the same stigma category:

> A category...can function to dispose its members to group-formation and relationships.[28]

The group or club may use a publication to share their feelings, and to give the reader a sense of belonging to the group:

> Here the ideology of the members is formulated - their complaints, their aspirations, their politics. The names of well-known friends and enemies of the 'group' are cited, along with information to confirm the goodness or the badness of these people. Success stories are printed, tales of heroes of assimilation who have penetrated new areas of normal

acceptance.[29]

So, written communication is a major theme in most such specialist groups, although a high level of literacy is not necessarily what one would expect of people in certain disadvantaged groups; the positive force of the newsletter may overcome the individual's usual disinclination to read and write:

> An intellectually worked-up version of their point of view is thus available to most stigmatised persons.[30]

Leaders of such groups are usually members of the stigmatised group, who emerge because of particular skills, qualities or dominant characteristics:

> Starting out as someone who is a little more vocal, a little better known, or a little better connected than his fellow-sufferers, a stigmatised person may find that the 'movement' has absorbed his whole day, and that he has become a professional.[31]

So, having become professional, they cross boundaries and deal with others outside their category of disadvantage. In the process they may well cease to be representative of the people whom they represent. Here, by way of illustration, Goffman uses what to some may be an irritating metaphor:

> Instead of leaning on their crutch, they get to play golf with it.[32]

The representative may, in addition to drawing closer to non-stigmatised people, also introduce their own slant on what is important or representative about the problem, and in this way too they may fail to represent the stigmatised group.

The other group of sympathisers are known as the Wise. These are people whose special situation makes them able to understand the stigmatised person, and gain acceptance by him or her. To become wise, the individual may have had to go through some personal process of becoming aware, and then they need to gain acceptance or validation by the stigmatised person or persons. Two broad groups make up the wise; the first is composed of professionals, for example nurses and other assistants working alongside stigmatised people such as criminals, homosexuals and prostitutes. The second is of those who acquire a special place because of a social relationship, through marriage, friendship or blood relationship. In this instance, the stigma has a tendency to spread to the other people in the relationship, such as, for example, the daughter of a convict.

**Moral career**

How a person comes to learn what is normal in society, how he or she comes to learn that he or she possesses a stigma, and what that means, this is a person's moral career. There are four patterns of moral career which may be experienced by stigmatised people:

- first, they may have an inborn stigma, such as a congenital deformity, and so they learn about their own stigmatised social identity simultaneously with learning about the norm;

- second, they may have an inborn stigma, but their protective family reduces the stigma, and maintains their feeling of normality until they are no longer able to be protected in this way - for example by going to school;

- third, they may acquire stigma late in life, perhaps because of illness or accident;

- and fourth, they may have been socialised elsewhere in the world, and have now come into a society where the norms are different.

The deviance from norms experienced by stigmatised persons is of those who aspire to the norm. So, there exists a 'normal-stigmatised unity,' which means that the person who becomes stigmatised in later life is not confused about their identity. They know very well what stigma means, having viewed it from the other side, from having been 'normal', the other side of 'interaction-uneasiness':

stigma involves...a pervasive two-role social process in which every individual participates in both roles, at least in some connections and in some phases of life.[33]

27

## Information control

Sometimes the stigmatised person is discredited, and at others he or she is only discreditable. On such occasions he or she faces a dilemma as to whether to display the stigma or not, thereby moving into the position of discredited person. As part of the process of transmitting information, the person will use a series of symbols, which convey social information. One such symbol would be a lapel badge which conveys information about club membership. Some symbols are prestige symbols, some are stigma symbols, while others (known as disidentifiers) break up an otherwise coherent picture.

Symbols, or signs, which act as prestige symbols are described as points, while those which convey stigma are described as slips. Some signs are incidental, and are not designed to transmit information. Others are designed to convey social information - for example badges, or military insignia. Some signs which originally were functional are now only informational, when their active function has now gone -such as behaviour to do with courtesy and etiquette. Others may be engineered to give information, although they present as functional - for example, duelling scars.

Signs may be congenital, permanent, or non-permanent. Non-permanent signs which have been inflicted against the will of the individual to convey social information are usually stigmatising.

A sign may mean one thing to one person or group, and something else to another - for example, the sign conveyed by a facial feature, or by a uniform. For this reason, and for others, signs are on occasions unreliable or misleading. Facial expressions may generally denote mood or temperament, but if they are induced by illness or mutilation, they are likely to have nothing to do with personality of the signifier.

Reference has already been made to the way in which the Own of a stigmatised person sometimes acquire an element of the same stigma, if they are related socially rather than professionally. This can be true of others who are not closely related, but who nonetheless associate with the stigmatised individual - the belief that who you are seen with tells people something about you, you are in some way contaminated by the same stigma - referred to as 'stigma by association.'

## Visibility and identification

How visible or otherwise evident a stigma is can be of great importance. Any change which can always be seen is crucial:

That which can be told about an individual's social identity at all times during his daily round and by all persons he encounters therein will be of great importance to him...any change in the way the individual must always and everywhere present himself will for these very reasons be fateful - this presumably providing the Greeks with the idea of stigma in the first place.[34]

The degree to which a visible stigma obtrudes will vary, and will depend not only on its objective extent, but also on the extent to which those who perceive it are able to understand its significance:

The decoding capacity of the audience must be specified before one can speak of degree of visibility.[35]

Although greater intimacy frequently overcomes prejudice and stigma, most people tend to maintain preconceptions about how they expect a person to behave, based on their social roles and on the social identity which has been ascribed to them. Evident stigma will be a contributor to this social identity. In the case of discreditable people, there is a constant fear that the person will be identified as having a stigma, even by close friends and members of the family. Indeed, the stigmatic feature may only become evident on closer acquaintance. It may be a feature of personal identity which only becomes an element of social identity when it is disclosed or discovered by others.

## Professional presentations

Goffman describes how a range of advice is offered by professionals and helpful others to stigmatised people on how to present in order to pass or cover. This includes the advice

- To develop a proper pattern for concealing and revealing;

- Never to pass completely;

- Never to accept the negative value of self which others impute to one;

- Not to 'minstrelise' - perform the part, or act the

29

clown;

-    And not to go to the other extreme, not to make too elaborate a statement about being normal.

Such advice, although sound and well meant, cannot fail to have the effect of making the person over-conscious of the situation in which they find themselves, and too detached. It also runs the risk of exposing very vulnerable, private areas of their lives.

On occasions, normal people express how stigmatised people should behave in relation to them in terms of being mature, well-adjusted, not concealing, but attempting to reach normal standards, without appearing to be completely normal, and excusing the tactlessness and hurt of normals to them:

> In many cases the degree to which normals accept the stigmatised individual can be maximised by his acting with full spontaneity and naturalness as if the conditional acceptance of him, which he is careful not to overreach, is full acceptance.[36]

If, however, he or she accepts fully what appears to be offered, there is embarrassment:

> ...every 'positive' relationship is conducted under implied promise of consideration and aid such that the relationship would be injured were these credits actually drawn on.[37]

## Style and meaning

Goffman's distinctive style, including his frequent use of metaphorical language, which was considered by John Lofland[38], requires some mention, in relation to *Stigma*. What Lofland refers to as 'perspective by incongruity'[39] is Goffman's deliberate use of expressions and concepts slightly removed from their usual context, requiring some redefinition of the terms which relate to the concept. For example, he will not make it clear whether he is using an expression as a literal statement or as a particular example of a more general point:

> Only a serious personal accident or the witnessing of a murder will create moments during these dead periods... [40]

30

The general point is made by stopping the reader short, and reflecting on the general point which must underlie the illustration. Elsewhere, the author makes his point in literal terms, but then shows that he was making a broader statement:

> ...stereotyping is classically reserved for customers, orientals, and motorists, that is, persons who fall into very broad categories... [41]

On other occasions, however, Goffman will express his theme only in figurative terms, most often by use of metaphor:

> ...her closet is as big as her beat, and she is the skeleton that resides in it.[42]

On occasions such as this, one wonders whether he has become at least as occupied with the niceness of style as with the meaning which he wishes to express. When this reaches the point of causing the reader to stop and consider the literary instrument, such as rhyme, rather than the concept behind it, style may have become the dominant issue:

> ...a case of revealing unsightedness while concealing unsightliness... [43]

But why does he do it? Is Goffman simply pre-occupied with his own cleverness? Lofland reminds us that the use of metaphor to attract and stimulate is no new strategy[44], and this could well be the principal purpose of such stylistic devices. However, part of the effect of the various forms of incongruity which he employs is to confuse: is this deliberate, or does Goffman miss the mark through his linguistic agility?

> The stigmatised person is almost always warned against attempting to pass completely. (After all, except for the anonymous confessor, it might be difficult for anyone to advocate this tack in open print.)[45]

In this instance, Goffman may be sharing with us an illustration which he has not developed and followed through, consequently rendering the whole point ambiguous; on the other hand he may be using an arresting example to make the point more sharply. Either way he confuses, as Lofland points out:

31

It is rather easy simply to misread his intentions. And, associated with misreading, is ambiguity in trying to pin down exactly what a given concept might mean.[46]

## Stigma and face

Facial disfigurement is an example of the primary meaning of stigma, as outlined by Goffman - a physical mark or stain. Stigma may also be experienced through the face arising from tribal or ethnic distinctiveness - being black, or looking Puerto Rican, are examples of this.

Facial appearance is also used to inform moral judgements about people whom we meet - we surmise that the other is a fighter, or a drinker, because of facial traits. This is deliberately invoked in order to illustrate a societal judgement on an offender - the sign of Cain, in Genesis, or the branding of a slave. In *Woman at the Edge of Time*,[47] Madge Piercy describes her idea of a new, humane, and enlightened world. Incarceration is eliminated, and instead, serious offenders are branded permanently on their brow to denote their status. This assures their continued integrated status, and at the same time sets them apart.

As early as 1955, Goffman was referring to the positive social rating which an individual holds about himself or herself as 'face'. *On Face-work*[48] was first published in 1955, and in it Goffman uses the word 'face' strictly in a metonymic sense of 'the positive social value a person effectively claims for himself by the line others assume he has taken during a particular contact'.[49] He refers to the common expressions associated with face which were alluded to during the introduction to this study, such as 'maintaining face' and 'losing face', giving them all strict definitions within the framework of his description of interaction. He emphasises that maintenance of face is not only the responsibility of the individual in question, but also that of the other party to the exchange: loss of face is embarrassing to the person who discredits as well as to the individual who has been discredited, and much energy will be spent on trying not to embarrass the individual.

This was reiterated in *Embarrassment and Social Organisation*[50] in 1956, when Goffman spoke of the 'embarrassment' of being discredited. This affected not only the person discredited, but also the person who had been tactless enough to cause the discomfort, and perhaps even others who had observed the interaction. Those who made claims, either deliberately or inadvertently, to a social position which they could not justify could render themselves isolated by their own embarrassment, because the only safe thing to do in the circumstances was to withdraw:

> Compromised in every encounter which he enters, he truly wears the leper's bell.[51]

The same theme is addressed and further developed in *The Presentation of Self in Everyday Life*,[52] when Goffman refers to the assumptions made by others about an individual, frequently before he or she speaks, and certainly thereafter, based on appearance, social position, and other factors external to the person.[53] This will be dealt with in further detail when discussing the contribution of Frances Macgregor, on whose anthropological work Goffman drew in *Stigma*.[54]

## Developments from Goffman's work

### Paul Hunt's Stigma

This is a series of views of stigma from the perspective of individual people with permanent physical disabilities -predominantly muscular dystrophy, rheumatoid arthritis and poliomyelitis.[55] The contributors all responded to letters from Hunt in national newspapers and magazines, and he himself contributed an article as well as publishing the anthology. All the authors are either describing their own experiences, or expressing views on disability which have derived directly from their own experiences.

Although stigma is the stated focus of the book, much of it is also concerned with wider aspects of disability - descriptions of how individuals managed to maintain near- normal living situations, the sadness of the disruption of family life, practical hints about survival, and strongly offered suggestions for developments and revisions of welfare services. On the question of stigma itself, two essays are of particular value, the first and the last.

The first, *The Chatterley Syndrome* by Louis Battye, considers Lawrence's novel[56] from the perspective of the paraplegic husband. Battye suggests that Lawrence is unable to suppress his distaste for Sir Clifford, whom he regards as less than human. This, he says, is largely society's view of the disabled person:

> And so, however he came to be in it, the cripple, the

physically underprivileged man, lives in his underprivileged sub-world, the world in which all his actions are strangely distorted and diminished in scale and significance, so that in some ways they seem like incompetent and slightly ridiculous parodies of the real thing.[57]

This is the 'felt stigma' referred to by Page below - whatever structures for care and welfare are constructed by society, this is what the individual experiences.

The final essay is by Hunt himself, in which he states that disabled people challenge society, and this for five reasons - because they are 'unfortunate, useless, different, oppressed and sick'. Disabled people are uncomfortable to be with:

For the able-bodied, normal world we are representatives of many of the things they most fear - tragedy, loss, dark and the unknown. Involuntarily we walk - or more often sit - in the valley of the shadow of death.[58]

These two contributions express powerfully the essence of stigma - the first tells us what it feels like, and the second offers an explanation of why we stigmatise which is very difficult to challenge.

*Paul Spicker's Stigma and Social Welfare*

Spicker's analysis[59] is concerned with the effect of stigma on those who receive social services. It aims[60] to clarify different uses of the expression 'stigma', to construct a coherent concept, and to consider the implications of the idea of stigma for social policy.

Spicker considers stigma as an attribute of the individual, pointing out that he has hitherto avoided defining it. He says that 'although the concept was born out of the social services, it cannot be understood in terms of the services alone'.[61] It was not born out of the social services; when the Greeks coined the expression, it had no suggestion of welfare; nor had the Christian mystics any notion of social services when they used the term to denote (in a most positive sense) the marks of the Crucifixion. Spicker's principal source for defining it as an individual attribute is Goffman, which he intersperses with more references to stigmatising welfare services, such as free school meals, thereby confusing the analysis.

Spicker's chapter on physical and mental stigmas (sic) could have been useful, but its value is reduced by a circular argument. The

34

author says that stigma is strongly associated with rejection, and thereafter uses the expressions inter-changeably. Then he states that there are at least three occasions for the rejection of physically stigmatised people. The first is that they tend to be poor, the second is that physical disability tends to cause dependence, and the third is because they can be disfigured. But disfigurement is the stigma - the stigma is stigmatising.[62]

The remainder of the work places the stigmatised individual in a social context. A useful reference is made to Watson when considering the immorality of being poor:

> Those who neglect their capacity and opportunity for self-help ... fail to display those abilities which make a human being worthy of respect ... [63]

Perhaps this helps us to understand why individual disfigured people join self-help groups: in order to overcome potentially negative judgement to which they are susceptible because of their disfigurement, they become visibly self- sufficient by participation in the group activity.

In summary, some stigmata occasion a lower status than others, and that status is determined by several factors. One of the most important factors is the way in which stigma may spiral because of the interaction between the individual and the rest of society - the individual is rejected because of his or her stigma, and so withdraws, thereby enhancing the stigma, and making more pronounced rejection likely. This is an important idea, but generally the book is disappointing and confusing.

*Robert Page's Stigma*

A much more coherent analysis of the relationship between stigma and welfare is offered by Robert Page,[64] in his *Stigma*, which was published in 1984, the same year as Spicker's work. Both were versions of the authors' doctoral theses. Page offers a framework for understanding stigma which is predominantly Goffman's, and so does not need to be restated in detail, but one point of relevance which he accentuates is that stigmata will attract varying levels of blame depending on their origin; generally, physical stigmata are less blameworthy than others, such as conduct stigmata, but even physical stigmata attract different amounts of censure; two factors which influence this are of particular importance - first, if the stigma has

35

been brought about by the individual (for example, many would say that obesity should be so censured), and second, if there is also present a moral stigma (such as criminality); this will over-ride the sympathy which the physical stigma might normally attract.

Yet despite the fact that not all stigmata are blamed on the individual, they are stigmata for all that, and continue to carry the tendency to down-grade the persons who carry them.

The remainder of Page's work is not material to this discussion; he considers a group of people, unmarried mothers, who have been stigmatised over centuries, in order to gain insights into why certain groups rather than others are stigmatised within contemporary society. The relationship is then discussed between stigma, justice and rights to receive welfare; finally, the use of stigma as a means of social control is discussed.

## Stigma and facial surgery

Goffman's explanation of the behaviour of stigmatised people, and of others in relation to stigmatised people, is illustrated by several facets of the present study. Most of the patients who were interviewed in the field study had evident scarring; those who did not frequently had other indicators of being different, which became evident when they spoke, or ate.

In addition, although it has not been possible to examine the psychological functioning of the patients, before and after treatment, it may be that those who were psychologically more stable were less likely to feel the effects of stigma. This is a dimension not addressed by Goffman, who considers stigma as an independent variable rather than as dependent on other influences and constraints. The reality is that many factors will influence the individual's adjustment to a stigmatised state.

In the relationship or encounter between stigmatised person and other, the stigmatised person will consume more energy, and feel more pain, than the other, normal, person. Goffman's focus is almost exclusively the problem which this presents to the stigmatised person; however, the other person, although it may not hurt as much, may have as much trouble behaving and speaking in such a way as to reduce the impact of the stigma. Goffman refers to the tendency of others to invade the privacy of stigmatised people, as a right. On the other hand, this could arise from the well-disposed other's wish to compensate for their aversion to the stigma, and to demonstrate their preparedness to associate with the stigmatised individual. Striking a balance between not invading privacy on the one hand, and showing acceptance of the stigmatised person on the other, is hard, and Goffman does not acknowledge that it is so for the 'normal' person:

> Presumably this will have larger consequences for the stigmatised, since more arranging will usually be necessary on their part.[65]

The present study illustrates Goffman's reference to the 'Own', those who are particularly sympathetic to the stigmatised group by virtue of sharing the stigma. Several mutual help groups are described in Chapter Six, which have been established by competent and articulate people who also possess a stigmatising characteristic. This founder or leader becomes the group's advocate, their negotiator with the broader society, but may well not be representative of the original group, since he or she has achieved what someone with such a stigma is not accustomed to achieve, television appearances, travelling scholarships, and respect from professional bodies.

On the matter of information control, it is important to note that those with a facial disfigurement have difficulty with passing. Using Goffman's constructs, they are more likely to 'cover', that is, reduce the harmful impact of a known stigma. Those with a facial stigma usually find it difficult or impossible to conceal completely; it can be disguised, camouflaged or corrected, but there is very often a residual blemish. Surgery may be good, but the result is usually only an approximation to the original, unblemished state, and its successful results are often measured in terms of what it has improved, rather than its having achieved a return to the original state. Some of the participants in the study had no evident mark, and it is to these that passing is an issue; their disfigured state would only be brought into the open if they, for example, began to speak, or some other less evident result of the illness or treatment was exposed. Those whose tongue or part of tongue had been removed, or who had had their larynx or pharynx removed, would have serious speech problems. In many instances these improved over time, sometimes with the assistance of the speech therapist, but most were left with a residual impairment. Those who were not often thought that they still sounded different, and remained self-conscious about speaking. Eating too was a problem for many, because of the removal of part of the mouth, and of the teeth in some cases. Difficulty was experienced in eating hard foods, and dribbling food or drink because of poor control caused severe embarrassment. Most resolved this by avoidance, that is they stayed at home and did not eat or drink except in the presence of very close acquaintances. So, 'passing' is not the most important issue; most of the patients did not attempt to present as normal. They either tried to reduce the impact of appearing abnormal, for example by camouflage or prosthesis, or they avoided the issue completely, concealing themselves by staying at home.

## Conclusions

1. The concept of social differentness to which censure or negative judgement is attached may be traced back to very early sources, including the Old Testament.

2. The deviance literature of the 1960s debated the concepts of 'normal' and 'abnormal', but did not clearly distinguish between abnormality due to appearance and abnormality due to behaviour. abnormal appearance does carry a stigma, as subsequent writers such as Hunt and Page verify. Goffman made a general plea for tolerance in *Stigma*, pointing out that ideas of normality are relative, and that virtually anyone in society may be stigmatised for something.

3. Goffman also developed the concept of 'spoiled identity', and explored ways in which people handle stigma - such as 'passing', 'covering', 'withdrawal', and fighting back. Some of these strategies are more appropriate than others for people with very evident stigma such as a facial deformity or disfigurement.

4. The question of stigma is more keen when dealing with strangers. Davis refers to the process of 'breaking through' when overcoming the initial resistance of strangers. Goffman qualifies this, but his argument is thin at this point.

5. The complete social context of the stigmatised person must be addressed when establishing the overall impact on the individual of his or her stigma.

6. Many of the concepts and analyses applied to stigma in general apply to people with facial disfigurement.

# Notes

1. Becker, H.S., (ed.), 1964, *The Other Side - Perspectives on Deviance*, Free Press, New York.
2. Schur, E., 1965, *Crimes Without Victims: deviant behaviour and public policy: abortion, homosexuality, drug addition*, Prentice-Hall, Englewood Cliffs, New Jersey.
3. Szasz, T., 1971, *The Manufacture of Madness*, R.K.P., London, referring to Leviticus, XIV, 7-10. The goat was usually shaved, to indicate its stigmatised status.
4. Erikson, K.T., 'Notes on the Sociology of Deviance,' in Becker, H.S., (ed.), 1962, *The Other Side*, a revision of a paper first published in Social Problems, Vol. 9 pp. 307-314.
5. op. cit., p. 15.
6. op. cit., p. 20.
7. op. cit., p. 11.
8. Macgregor, F.C., 1974, *Transformation and Identity*, Quadrangle/New York Times Book Company, New York.
9. Bull, R., 1983, 'The General Public's Reaction to Facial Disfigurement', presented at the conference on *The Psychology of Cosmetic Treatment*, University of Pennsylvania, Philadelphia.
10. Goffman, E., 1963, *Stigma - Notes on the Management of Spoiled Identity*, Prentice-Hall, Englewood Cliffs, published 1968, Pelican, Harmondsworth.
11. Goffman, E., 1961, *Asylums*, Anchor Books, New York. 1968, Penguin, Harmondsworth.
12. Greenblatt, M., and Lindz, T., 1957, 'Some Dimensions of the Problem,' *The Patient and the Mental Hospital*, Greenblatt, M., Levinson, D.J., and Williams, R.H., Glencoe, Free Press.
13. Goffman, op.cit., p. 11.
14. op.cit., p. 21.
15. op.cit., p. 23.
16. op.cit., p. 94.
17. op.cit., p. 95.
18. ibid.
19. op.cit., p. 110.
20. op.cit., p. 127.
21. op.cit., p. 28.
22. op.cit., p. 30.
23. op.cit., p. 52.

24. Davis, F., 1961-2, 'Deviance Disavowal: the Management of Strained Interaction by the Visibly Handicapped,' *Social Problems*, 9, pp. 120-132.

25. Partridge, J., 1990, *Changing Faces - The Challenge of Facial Disfigurement*, Penguin, Harmondsworth, p. 67.

26. Goffman, op. cit., p. 53.

27. ibid.

28. op.cit., p. 36.

29. op.cit., p. 37.

30. op.cit., p. 38.

31. ibid.

32. op.cit., p. 39.

33. p. 163.

34. op.cit., p. 65.

35. op.cit., p. 68.

36. op.cit., p. 148.

37. ibid.

38. Lofland, J., 1980, 'Early Goffman: Style, Structure, Substance, Soul', *The View from Goffman*, ed. Jason Ditton, Macmillan, London.

39. Lofland, op.cit., p. 25, following Kenneth Burke, 1936, *Permanence and Change*, New Republic Inc., New York.

40. Goffman, op.cit., p. 89.

41. op.cit., p. 68.

42. op.cit., p. 99.

43. op.cit., p. 126.

44. op.cit., p. 25.

45. op.cit., p. 133.

46. op.cit, p. 27.

47. Piercy, M., 1978, *Woman on the Edge of Time*, Women's Press, London.

48. Goffman,E., 1955, 'On Face-Work: An Analysis of Ritual Elements in Social Interaction', *Psychiatry*, Vol. 18, No. 3, pp. 213-231, August, repeated in 1967, *Interaction Ritual: Essays on Face-to-Face Behaviour*, Doubleday Anchor, New York.

49. ibid., p. 5.

50. Goffman, E., 1956, 'Embarrassment and Social Interaction', *American Journal of Sociology*, Vol. 62, No. 23, November, pp. 264-271, printed in Goffman, E., 1967, *Interaction Ritual: Essays on Face-to-Face Behaviour*, Doubleday Anchor, New York.

51. ibid., p. 106.

52. Goffman,E., 1959, *The Presentation of Self in Everyday Life*,Doubleday Anchor, New York.

53. Although *The Presentation of Self in Everyday Life* was published in 1959, it had its origins in an earlier edition, published at the University of Edinburgh, in 1956, emphasising Goffman's anthropological base, since much of 'The Presentation' draws on anthropological observations made during fieldwork in the Shetlands, while Goffman was based in Edinburgh.

54. See for example Macregor,F. et al., 1953, *Facial Deformities and Plastic Surgery*, Charles C. Thomas, Springfield, Ill.

55. Hunt, P.(ed.), 1966, *Stigma: the Experience of Disability*, Chapman, London.

56. Lawrence, D.H., 1960, *Lady Chatterley's Lover*, Penguin, Harmondsworth.

57. Battye, L., 'The Chatterley Syndrome', in Hunt, op. cit., p. 15.

58. Hunt, P., 'A Critical Condition,' in Hunt, op. cit., p. 155.

59. Spicker, P., 1984, *Stigma and Social Welfare*, Croom Helm, Beckenham.

60. op. cit., p. 4.

61. op. cit., p. 61.

62. op. cit., p. 71.

63. Watson, D., 1980, *Caring for Strangers: an Introduction to Practical Philosophy for Students of Social Administration*, R.K.P., London, p. 57.

64. Page, R., 1984, *Stigma*, R.K.P., London.

65. Goffman, *Stigma*, p. 23.

# 2 An anthropological view

The contribution of Frances Cooke Macgregor to the study of facial disfigurement is unique. It spans forty years, and it has its origins in anthropology. Professor Macgregor's earliest work was an anthropological study of North American Indians. In the process of this study, some photographic work was required. A reconstructive surgeon named John Marquise Converse was put in touch with her, as he required the services of a specialist photographer in order to chart his work of facial reconstruction. Frances Macgregor was therefore introduced to the subject, and brought a range of skills to what became broadly a sociological approach to the subject.

In the course of her academic career Frances Macgregor conducted four major empirical studies. These are summarised below. In addition, she has published several theoretical works which derived from the field work. She has also contributed several articles which apply her findings to the situations of professionals - social workers, surgeons and lawyers, in particular.

*Social and psychological studies of plastic surgery*,[1] provides a useful summary of research into social and psychological factors associated with plastic surgery, and comments on the state of research on the subject over the previous 30 years.

When Professor Macgregor began her work in the late 1940s, and for the next 20 years, the emphasis generally was on the study of those requiring elective, cosmetic surgery, rather than of those severely deformed who required reconstruction. Plastic surgeons were looking for indications of those patients who might react in a negative manner post- operatively.

For many years, there was a focus on 'individual psychology and intrapsychic issues, to the exclusion of interpersonal and social reality factors'.[2] Plastic surgeons were still relying on the opinions of psychiatrists and clinical psychologists to inform their judgements of

43

the suitability of patients, although the part played by social and cultural factors in satisfaction with results had become more evident.

The other related research area which expanded over the period focused on the part played by beauty in social acceptance:

> We now have a substantial and growing body of research documenting the profound effects of physical attractiveness and unattractiveness in social perception, personality assessments, behavioural expectations, and human interaction.[3]

This underlines the value and importance of aesthetic plastic surgery, which is more than just a pursuit for the vain.

The main defect at that point, according to Professor Macgregor, was in the area of longitudinal studies. This remains the case to this day. Presumably she was not including herself completely in this, as she had by then made a substantial contribution by virtue of her 1979 work.[4]

## Empirical studies

The first of her empirical studies, reported in 1950, was carried out in the late 1940's; Macgregor and Schaffner[5] looked at a group of 73 applicants for nose reduction or alteration, in order to understand first, the characteristics of those who seek nose operations, second, what were the factors which would cause the clinical team to proceed or reject the application, and third, what were the factors which determine patient satisfaction with the results.[6]

The patients were aged 13 to 43; 39 were male and 34 were female. Fifty-nine of them were unmarried. After the clinical history had been obtained by the surgeon, the patients were then seen by the research interviewer, for anything from three to ten one-hour sessions. Initially, the real reasons for wanting surgery were often concealed, and only later admitted. Five case histories are presented, two of people who were recommended for surgery, and three where it was contra-indicated.

The reasons for wishing for surgery were partly social, and partly psychological. The social reasons were:

    i.    to overcome an economic or social handicap;
    ii.    to subscribe to the cultural norms of beauty;
    iii.    to eliminate the cause of ridicule;

iv.     to gain approval and enhance the self-concept;
v.      to avoid people pre-judging the character;
vi.     to obtain full membership of a social group;
vii.    to cross caste or class lines, and
viii.   to avoid racial stereotype.

The psychological reasons were:

i.      to alter the personality;
ii.     to correct psychological difficulties;
iii.    to reduce feelings of inferiority;
iv.     to be popular;
v.      to improve relationships;
vi.     to avoid facing more profound problems;
vii.    to remove a trait which is also owned by a parent who
        has rejected the patient;
viii.   to gain dependency or closeness to others;
ix.     to prove that he or she has no fear of pain;
x.      to explain or account for a failure in life, and
xi.     to change identity.

Traits found which were viewed as contra-indications were:

i.      vague explanations;
ii.     a defect smaller than the patient suggests;
iii.    a defect which is lesser than another, more noticeable
        defect;
iv.     excessive or obscure expectations;
v.      where surgical improvements will not be able to match
        the hopes of the patient;
vi.     where the patient is psychologically unready;
vii.    where the pressure for surgery is from other people;
viii.   where previous operations have failed to satisfy
ix.     hypochondriasis;
x.      a history of maladjustment;
xi.     where the patient blames external forces for the course
        of his or her life, and
xii.    when there has been a previous psychiatric disorder.

These typologies were composed almost forty years ago, and
consequently some of them may seem slightly dated; to cite a previous
psychiatric disorder as grounds for not proceeding with surgery could

today be seen as an infringement of civil rights. Nonetheless they are a useful starting point, and many of the pointers which they provide are still topical and relevant.

The second empirical study is described by Macgregor et al., of 1953.[7] The chapter written by Frances Macgregor describes the impact of plastic surgery on the lives of 74 patients, and the extent of their satisfaction with the work of the surgeons. (She also draws out several general lessons learned from the field work, and these are summarised later in this chapter.) Of the 74 patients studied, 32 had completed or almost completed surgery, and all but one were highly or fairly pleased. The remaining one was seeking further surgery, and was highly discontented with the results. No personality changes were noted following surgery, but many patients noted changes in their social performance:

> As for the patients themselves, feelings of shame, self-consciousness, inferiority, and social inadequacy were mitigated, and there was a marked rise in self- esteem and self-confidence. Many felt that they 'no longer stood out from the crowd' but 'looked normal' or 'just like the next person'.[8]

Changes noted by the interviewers were:

> The behaviour of others improved because the subjects themselves had become more relaxed and tolerant;

> General appearance (clothing, carriage and manner) also improved;

> Energy previously used in preoccupation with the disfiguring condition was released to positive ends;

> Although basic personality did not change, negative character traits seemed to reduce in dimension.

Five case histories are given, showing the positive developments for each individual following surgery. One of these, a woman, underwent nasal reconstruction, and the following is an extract from her Sentence Completion Test, applied before and after surgery:[9]

46

| PREOPERATIVE | POSTOPERATIVE |
|---|---|
| Nicknames: 'Schnozzle Nose', 'Rummy' | Nicknames: Gone |
| Men: Stay to myself to avoid teasing | Men: Say what a change |
| Teasing is: Hourly | Teasing is: Over |
| Strangers: Avoid | Strangers: Not annoyed by their actions anymore |
| I envy: Just to be normal like the other fellow | I envy: No one |
| I become embarrased: because it is constant - no let up | I become embarrased: Not the but of a joke anymore |
| I like best: To be out of sight of strange people | I like best: My new nose |

In summary, although surgery is not the only or a certain way of improving mental health for facially disfigured people, nonetheless it may

> ... effect a reduction in feelings of hopelessness, isolation, and fear of people, and on the other hand promote or restore feeling of belonging and self- esteem.[10]

This study was also described preliminarily by Frances Macgregor in a paper given in 1951.[11] The article is a combination of general observations, statistical data and case histories. It describes the study as the first part of a longitudinal study. The format for data collection is not described, but it is stated that the number of interviews varied from patient to patient, ranging from three to 15 interviews. Although some statistical features are included, the interviews appear to have been of a semi-structured nature, allowing a full descriptive case history to be provided. It would have been interesting to have seen more hard data, in order to justify in a quantitative way some of the statements made. However, it must be remembered that the author is using observational methods which are anthropological in origin - hence the numerous interviews, the actual numbers of which varied from person to person.

Feelings of belonging and self-esteem were very much the theme of her 1967 paper,[12], in which she described some features of 89 patients interviewed between 1946 and 1964 in New York City, who had presented for rhinoplasty, nose alteration. This is the third empirical study.

All those who were interviewed felt that surgery could help them, saying that their nose was currently a social impediment. Half were male, half were female. A quarter were under 20, and half were in their twenties. Seventy-two per cent were single. It cannot be said that the sample is necessarily socially representative, as most of the patients were drawn from a voluntary clinic. What is highly significant is their immigrant status:

### Table 2.1
### Frances Macgregor's 1967 Sample    N = 89
### (figures given are percentages)

| | % |
|---|---|
| First-generation American | 9 |
| Second-generation American | 63 |
| Third-generation American | 15 |
| Old White American | 3 |
| Negro American | 1 |
| Non-United States citizen | 7 |
| Not ascertained | 2 |

Thirty-nine per cent were of Jewish origin, 25% Italian, and 10% Eastern European. Forty-five per cent were Catholic, and 34% professed Judaism (a small number of Jewish origin had repudiated their parents' religion).

When considering why such a group requested rhinoplasty, the author stresses that social factors are at least as important as intrapsychic issues.

> To slide over the role that social and cultural factors may play in determining the wish for surgery and to concentrate on the more deeply rooted psychiatric factors is to obscure and by implication to oversimplify two other important dimensions: the relationship between the patient and his social and cultural milieu, and the extent to which the values of our society bring

pressure to bear on its members to conform.[13]

Most patients had been stared at, ridiculed and abused, resulting in feelings of inferiority and shame. They had difficulties in getting jobs and making friends.  Half wanted their noses changed for ethnic reasons - because they were associated with their origins, which they felt caused them to be down-trodden or held back socially or economically:

> These persons wanted to 'look like an American,' a statement to which some Jews added, 'I want a turned-up Irish nose.' In other words, they were primarily dissatisfied with their noses as visible cues to an ethnic or religious group that they perceived as having negative or stigmatic connotations. Surgery was viewed as a device by which they could eliminate this trait.[14]

The other half were motivated by wishing to avoid being stereotyped because of their nose - frequently being seen as a fighter, or ridiculed as being ugly. They wanted to be seen for what they were, rather than what they looked like.

For both groups the nose has become a disability irrespective of whether there is any functional impairment. How far this is so varies from society to society, and also varies over time. It is reasonable to argue that this group, being largely the children and grand children of immigrants, did not have the same need to cling to the characteristics of their ethnic origins, and wished instead to assimilate the characteristics of the dominant group in the United States.

Frances Macgregor concludes by suggesting that some of the elements of her study would provide valuable material for those currently engaged in the development of deviance theory, such as Becker, Davis and Goffman. As it happens, some of her early material is quoted by Goffman in *Stigma*. Both Frances Macgregor and Goffman were recipients of research grants from the National Institute for Mental Health in the 1950s, and it is therefore reasonable to suppose that Goffman and Frances Macgregor had some practical association during the period.

The fourth empirical work,[15] published in 1979, is a follow-up study of 16 of the 71 patients previously studied, 20 years on, published in 1979.  They were approached personally, and all who were approached agreed to be seen. Eight were male and eight were female; nine of the patients had originally been markedly disfigured, and seven grossly disfigured; 11 had congenital disfigurements, and five were acquired. Nine of the patients had moved to slightly or moderately disfigured. Of the seven grossly affected, five had reduced to marked, and one of the marked had deteriorated to gross because of ill-advised surgery.

Fourteen were now married; there was a tendency for members of the group to marry into a lower social class, and to accept anyone who would have them (or so they perceived it). There was a strong tendency (11) to be concerned with helping disadvantaged people, often with reference to disfigurement or disability.

Generally, the 16 had adjusted satisfactorily. Six illustration are provided in depth, showing how they had managed to cope with disfigurement. Some had become exceptionally skilful in social intercourse, while others had withdrawn for a substantial period. Most were now leading circumscribed lives, treating home as something of a refuge.

Most commonly, their strategy for survival had been denial, either that they had a handicap, or that it was as substantial as it actually was. Most of this denial was positive and useful:

> Although denial may be carried to lengths verging on pathological, the evidence in these cases is that it can be a desirable and helpful mechanism when it wards off anxiety and provides protection and a sense of mastery.[16]

All the interviewees showed a strong motivation to be recognised, to be 'someone', in spite of their disability. Yet they were still very vulnerable about their appearance, and angry and bitter because they had had to accept second best.

The fact that they achieved greater stability than the predictions made at the outset may suggest that the psychiatrists had taken an over-pathological view. A psychiatrist who carried out some of the original screening commented:

> We were not good judges of the degree to which individuals marshalled their strengths because of the fact that they have a reality disfigurement which is continually being reaffirmed.[17]

This suggested that the it was possible to mitigate the impact of the disfigurement by careful preparation and sensitivity when speaking to the disfigured person:

Since they can almost always count on a negative response wherever they go, they tend to be prepared and to develop overt or covert techniques of coping. Thus, predictability and consistency of response seem to be crucial factors that permit severely handicapped individuals to adjust, in contrast to the erratic nature and unpredictability of responses toward those with slight or moderate defects.[18]

The heaviest strain over the years was the management of the disfigured child in the family, and there was evidence of poor family functioning, with the child's brothers and sisters being badly affected - inconsistent or apparently unfair handling, over-protectiveness of the affected child, and the feeling of shame which hung over the family. There were some extreme examples of strain, which did not however cause complete breakdown:

> ... total rejection by a parent - and by total I mean to the extent that one parent left the home and completely abandoned the child at an early age - while having a crippling effect did not appear to be as devastating psychologically for the child as it might have been had the parent remained in the home.[19]

A general point was about the nature of disfigured people as a group and as individuals, which explained some of the special difficulty which they encounter:

> ... although highly visible as individuals, as a group the disfigured are invisible. Not only do they avoid public exposure; they do not colonise. They also eschew the kinds of self-help groups that now exist for almost every conceivable category of physical, psychological and social pathology.[20]

This is no longer true, as the present study describes, but the general point remains true: that the disfigured person faces an hostile environment, and it requires special courage to overcome it, with the consequence that many stay hidden or semi-hidden, as this study shows.

## Sociological lessons

### A social handicap

Frances Macgregor's paper in The American Sociological Review in 1951[21] describes the person with a facial disfigurement as having a social and an economic handicap rather than one of physical functioning, as the face has paramount significance:

> It is the source of vocal communication, the expression of emotions, and the revealer of personality traits. The face is the person himself.[22]

Assumptions are made about a person at first encounter, which may or may not be borne out by longer acquaintance; these assumptions are based largely on appearance. Someone who has the facial characteristics of a disadvantaged or stigmatised group is therefore set apart. For example, those with congenital deformity are stared at and mocked as freaks - certain types of facial contour are associated with character traits, such as the weak chin with unreliable character.

Facially disfigured people are aware of these pre- dispositions, and consequently react disproportionately strongly to the disfigurement itself. This is particularly so when the preconceptions are taken to the point of a stereotype held about people of certain facial types - 'social or cultural stereotyping.' The facial shape is associated with character type, usually negatively, and frequently this has a disproportionately serious impact on the individual.

> Such misconceptions and interpretations seem to play a significant part in the self-regarding attitudes and subsequent development of psychological conflicts in many of the facially deformed.[23]

How the deformity has originated may determine the acceptance or non-acceptance of the person - this is the fifth pressure referred to by Frances Macgregor. If it is believed to have been acquired in a socially unacceptable way, judgements are made, frequently erroneously - for example, if the deformity is believed to have been acquired in a fight, the bearer is seen as the sort of person who gets into fights, whether he or she has been disfigured in that manner, or in some other way, such as an accident, or cancer. Moreover, if cancer is believed to be the cause, the same veil of silence is drawn over the result as clothes the illness itself.

Linked with this is the issue of social expectancy. As a controlled trial at the University of New York showed (carried out in conjunction with Professor Macgregor's project), facial appearance plays a major part in forming views about the person. For example, comments about a man whose face had been burned and who then contracted facial cancer included:

> 'Probably a gangster.'
> 'Horrible!'
> 'Grotesque, inhuman, bad.'
> 'A leper.'[24]

Again, a man with a congenital deformity was described:

> 'He is mean and small - not bright. His worst problem is a slightly abnormal receding chin.'
> 'He looks mean and nasty.'
> 'He might be a follower in a gang.'
> 'He's a dope addict.'
> 'I wouldn't hire him for a job where he would meet people because I think his appearance is against him.'
> 'Man seems to look like a maniac. Has desire to kill.'
> 'Below average intelligence - probably an I.Q. slightly above or even in moron group.'
> 'Repulsive because of deformed teeth.'
> 'Appears to be an imbecile; very low intelligence'.[25]

In fact, this man was a junior executive in a chemical firm. Presumably he is thought to be a follower in a gang because his receding chin precludes him from leadership.

The other side of the same phenomenon is that society may ascribe all behavioural difficulties to the facial disorder -the pressures on the disfigured person are real, but they do not necessarily induce pathological behaviour.

In *Transformation and Identity*[26] Frances Macgregor drew together her research experience in order to formulate a series of theoretical concepts. One of its most important contributions is that in it Frances Macgregor offers a definition of disfigurement:

> ... facial deformity is defined as any physical deviation that differentiates the victim from others to the extent that it may be

regarded as socially or psychologically handicapping.[27]

Strangely, the definition does not mention 'face', but its importance is that deformity is not defined in terms of physical attribute, but of intra- and inter-personal context.

There are several strong links with Goffman in this work - Frances Macgregor refers to 'civil inattention':

> The 'civil inattention' that strangers normally confer on one another and that makes it possible to move unhindered in pub lic places and to conduct one's affairs without fear of personal intrusion is denied the disfigured person.[28]

## The significance of parts of the face

A caution is expressed by the author[29] that small imperfections should be taken seriously, and that one should not concentrate wholly on major disorders. The face is a sensitive medium, and any impairment of expression will impede communication. She underlines this statement by concluding with a quotation from Goffman:

> The closer the defect is to the communication equipment upon which the listener must focus his attention, the smaller the defect needs to be to throw the listener off balance. These defects tend to shut off the afflicted individual from the stream of daily contacts, transforming him into a faulty interactant, either in his own eyes or in the eyes of others.[30]

## Societal reactions

Facial disfigurement is a handicap, not because of functional impairment, but because of the impact of societal attitude on the person - a psychosocial problem. Ten years before Goffman's *Stigma*, Frances Macgregor described the significance of 'visibility:

> Once the standards of normality and abnormality are determined - in this case what constitutes an attractive face or an ugly one - we must recognise the important role of visibility as it functions in the interactional processes between the disfigured individual and those with whom he comes in

contact.[31]

First impressions of the individual derive from the perception of the face - even if they are subsequently adjusted by a learned tolerance:

> The individual with an unfavourable physical trait, therefore, may be the object of an immediate negative reaction even though it may be followed by the recognition that sympathy should have been the feeling awakened by his condition.[32]

Whether or not the face is unsightly, it may be misleading, disguising the real person, or the finer thoughts or feelings usually illustrated through facial expression. The disfigured individual is constrained by the deformity from participating fully in social roles. This chapter explains what the constraints are, and how disfigured people adjust to them. It then describes the social outcomes of a study of facial plastic surgery - the impact on the individuals and their lives.

## The impact of small blemishes

The high value given to facial attractiveness operates against disfigured people. Frances Macgregor refers to her first major study, in which the characteristics of 115 people with a range of facial disfigurement were interviewed over a three-year period, in the process of which she found that:

> ... the severity of the disfigurement had no direct proportional relationship to the degree of psychic distress it engendered nor the kinds of adjustments made to it.[33]

## Ridicule

The theme of the significance of small blemishes links with the question of ridicule. In her 1970 article referred to above, the author makes the point that those with a minor facial defect are also more likely to be laughed at than those with a severe impairment, who may well evoke pity. Ridicule or laughter can be most punitive; she cites the Hopi Indians, who drive enemies away by laughing at them. Even minor impairment must be taken seriously, particularly in the area around the mouth, which is so emotionally charged and evocative.

55

The issue of ridicule is discussed in an early study, when the group reported being ridiculed, being stared at, and being rejected, but there were also very tangible problems over getting jobs, friends and partners, with the resultant psychological distress and disturbances sometimes becoming quite severe; reactions ranged from feelings of inferiority to psychotic states.[34]

Frances Macgregor[35] described how minor facial anomalies in children, only severe enough to cause ridicule, had a more serious emotional impact on the child than disfigurement which evoked pity or aversion. Children always ridicule ear anomalies, and this may cause lasting emotional harm. To avoid this, corrective surgery should be carried out as early as possible, to ensure acceptance by the peer group. Although the child may not complain, nonetheless they are likely to be very bothered. There appears to be little gender differentiation - girls are just as bothered as boys, although they may camouflage their disfigurement partially by means of long hair.

## The significance of beauty

A further factor which works against disfigured people is the heavy emphasis placed on physical attractiveness, and upon conformity to what a particular society holds to be the norm for attractiveness:

> Every culture has its own standards of attractiveness, and while an infinite number of physical divergencies are possible which meet the aesthetic requirements, a certain conformity is demanded.[36]

If isolation is to be avoided, so must differentness.

Because the first impression caused by the facial appearance is what encourages or repels further social interaction, the disfigured person is placed at a substantial disadvantage when trying to make relationships:

> As far as social stimuli are concerned, probably greater differentiation is made in human society between the physically attractive and the unattractive people than is drawn between the sexes ... a handsome person, regardless of what he may say or do, tends to evoke responses that are not what they would be were he ugly.[37]

## Ethnicity

During the early days of Professor Macgregor's work, there was a strong emphasis in the United States on conforming to the norm of American appearance. Whether or not this was defined, non-conformity was often evident - if one looked excessively Jewish, for example, or Armenian; her subsequent writing shows how transient these cultural stereotypes are- a generation on and those asking for nose reduction were trying to look Irish - like the Kennedy family. One wonders whether now the culture has gone full circle, with the increased pride in origins, be they European, African or Asian.[38]

## Myths

A whole range of beliefs and myths exists about the origins of facial blemishes and disfigurement; even if few would admit to believing them wholeheartedly, as with much superstition, many find them hard to discount completely. Broadly, they are either associated with primitive myths (such as contact with a hare) or they are associated with the wrath of God for wrongdoing.[39]

## Strategies for managing

All of the patients in this study developed strategies for lessening the tension which the disfigurement caused - withdrawal, aggression, blaming others, and partial or complete denial of the disfigurement. Similarly, techniques were developed for managing difficulties encountered in public:

> To be the object of curiosity, furtive looks, manifestations of pity, ridicule, or repulsion, is to feel conspicuous and different. [40] (Here is an early reference to 'shameful differentness'.)

How disfigured people responded to this was not determined by the extent of their disfigurement, but rather by the distinctive features of their personality, or by the nature of the social situation. Some might turn away, others disguise themselves, others stare back, or become otherwise hostile, some joke, some deliberately create situations which give others the chance to get used to the disfigurement.

In Professor Macgregor's first major study, from 1946-1949, of 115 plastic surgery patients,[41] she describes the major difficulties as being with employment, friends, marriage and general discrimination. There were also problems with staring, remarks, laughter, intrusive questioning, and eye avoidance. She described the strategies used, which included remaining aloof, avoiding certain forms of social activity, seclusion, aggression, blaming others, and using the deformity itself as a defence and justification for disturbance. It was also found that many patients adjusted by denying that the problem was as great as it manifestly was.

## Dissatisfaction with surgery

Macgregor and Ford[42] considered the phenomenon of the dissatisfied plastic surgery patient; some of the dissatisfaction is justified, resulting from incompetent practice, but some is due to the fact that the surgeon does not investigate sufficiently the motivation of the individual for seeking surgery. Apparently trivial motives may be important - for example, the removal of a visible scar may be to remove the social slur which the scar implies; generally speaking, the surgeon is advised to be more wary of those who seek the correction of minor defects than major, and especially of those with unrealistic expectations of the impact which surgery will make - black people who feel that their ethnic origin will be disguised by a different shape may unconsciously be hoping to be made white.

This is not to diminish the value of corrective surgery, which has dramatic effects on the personal functioning of many patients, but it does not affect the underlying personality:

> ... only the functioning of the patient's personality, not his underlying personality, is affected. Underneath a new nose schizophrenics remain schizophrenics, neurotics neurotics.[43]

Mental illness in itself is no bar, as long as there is clarity of motivation, and the authors provide a very vivid example of a successful outcome of rhinoplasty to a 28-year-old woman with schizophrenia, whose underlying condition remained, despite evident satisfaction at the physical and social consequences of surgery.

Frances Macgregor explores the theme in more depth in an article in Aesthetic Plastic Surgery in 1981.[44] She looks at two groups of causes of dissatisfaction amongst patients whose surgery is apparently satisfactory.

The first group of causes of dissatisfaction are those which relate to the patients themselves:

- psychological problems;
- they hoped that surgery would resolve other life difficulties;
- they had unrealistic expectations of what surgery would achieve;
- they were subjected to external pressures to have surgery;
- they were too dependent on others for the achievement of their self-esteem.

The surgeon was also deemed to be responsible for the dissatisfaction in a number of situations, as described below:

- he or she had made a hasty evaluation;
- the patient had not been prepared for what to expect;
- what was involved had been minimised;
- the surgeon was doing what he or she thought was the best thing;
- the surgeon did not listen empathetically.

In other instances again, there could be said to be faults on both sides - a personality clash, or simply poor communication by both the surgeon and the patient.

In all, the most common reason for outcome dissatisfaction is failure to interview properly. For example, the surgeon may make assumptions about what the patient wants, instead of asking; he or she may, for example, make cultural assumptions which are not transferable to the culture of the interviewee.

A very practical caution is expressed about secondary scars; quite simply they need to be kept to an unavoidable minimum; they are a mutilation which is not expected, and therefore may be very damaging to the individual.

## Plastic surgeons

Patient dissatisfaction is good for neither patient nor surgeon - the patient has to endure lasting unsightliness and unhappiness, and the doctor the criticism of his or her work, sometimes resulting in litigation. Although one may deplore the litigiousness which attaches to surgery, it is a reality, and practical steps must be taken to minimise the risk, for the sake of everyone. Running right through Macgregor's advice to surgeons is the clear, simple message: open, honest communication is the best prevention of law suits. This has been reinforced by conversations which the author has had with surgeons in the United Kingdom and in North America.

In a lecture given to the American Academy of Ophthalmology and Otolaryngology in 1951,[45] a description is offered of the psychological consequences of facial disfigurement, which may be harder to remove than the physical defect. The activity of the surgeon may have a direct impact on both, but on occasions the amount of felt improvement in appearance is not proportionate either to the original disorder or the amount of physical improvement achieved by surgery. Macgregor warned that when deciding whether to offer surgery the reconstructive surgeon should investigate:

1)   The motives behind the request;
2)   The patient's reason for wanting the operation at this particular time;
3)   The patient's expectations as to the cosmetic and subjective result.[46]

This may not come easily to the surgeon; the literature describes surgeons as keen to act to solve complex practical and technological problems, with little emphasis on good communication with their patients. But in the matter of facial reconstruction, the relationship between surgeon and patient affects recovery and rehabilitation, and difficulties which the patient may make (non-co-operation, anger, vacillation) will be construed by the surgeon as dispositional, rather than situational. The surgeon must acknowledge cultural and social class differences, and level of education of the patient, given that:

... the patient who is given a thorough explanation throughout the stages of his treatment not only tends to participate more actively and effectively with the surgeon but is more likely to accept the plans and goals for rehabilitation.[47]

The surgeon should be conscious of his or her motivation in offering treatment; excessive zeal to create beauty, often referred to as the 'Pygmalion complex,' may obscure the fact that the patient does not want the operation as much as the doctor does; dissatisfaction with the result becomes a strong possibility.

The surgeon is concerned in his or her day-to-day work with the activity of the operating room, rather than with direct communication with the patient - surgeons tend to be people of action, regarding technical problems as a challenge. This poses a problem:

> In reality, however, success in management, treatment and rehabilitation of the disfigured patient is determined in no small measure by the kind of relationship established between him and his doctor.[48]

The doctor needs to be prepared for a range of people and reactions, which will not always be positive. Reasons for negative reactions to surgery are usually sociological or cultural, rather than intra-psychic - this is the constant theme of Macgregor the anthropologist. Two valuable case illustrations reinforce the point.

The general rule, to avoid all misunderstanding, dissatisfaction and litigation is:

> ... that the patient who is given a thorough explanation throughout the stages of his treatment tends not only to participate more actively and effectively with the surgeon but is more likely to accept the plans and goals for rehabilitation.[49]

By this stage in her research career, Frances Macgregor was able to offer very clear, authoritative precepts to surgeons:

- To have care when discussing technical matters in front of patients;
- Not to withhold facts for which patients should be prepared;
- Not to say that the disfigurement is less than it is;
- Always to discover how much patients are expecting;
- To talk to and listen to the patient.

**The patient-surgeon relationship**

In one of her later works,[50] the author discusses the relationship which needs to exist between patient and surgeon if successful rehabilitation is to be completed. She is referring in particular to reconstructive surgery where a loss has occurred resulting from trauma or cancer, and begins by reviewing the impact which such a loss will necessarily have upon the individual.

Surgeons and other clinical staff must therefore ensure that the patient understands fully the restorative process - what it can and cannot do, and how long it will take.

> Throughout the often long and complicated struggle toward total rehabilitation, a high degree of motivation is essential. To help the patient maintain it, the support and understanding of the surgeon, staff, relatives, and friends are of inestimable value. Essential also to achieving optimal results in a long-term rehabilitation program is the co-operative effort of patient and surgical team.[51]

## Openness

Not everyone's idea of a good result is the same, and the surgeon should go through every detail of the possible outcomes of surgery, to ensure that the patient understands it, and fully wants it in all respects:

> The surgeon should insist on as much specificity as possible from patients about what they want or don't want done and why, and in turn explain as definitively as he can what alterations he has in mind.[52]

A 1976 article[53] focuses on pitfalls for plastic surgeons, who must be careful in their choice of patient, for their own sake and that of their patient:

> ... systematic studies of persons seeking plastic surgery show that care in interviewing and evaluating those with minimal defects is of far more critical importance than it is with those who are markedly disfigured.[54]

Generally, the precept was to listen to and with the patient, and see everything in context. Macgregor includes a lengthy illustrative interview, showing the contraindications for surgery. In the long run, the surgeons did carry out the requested procedure referred to in the illustration, and the patient was dissatisfied and bitter.

## Seeing the patient as a whole

Full acknowledgement should be made of the patient's identity, and he should not be treated simply as an object. Reference is made to the practice of discussing a patient in the latter's presence, without full interpretation of the discussion to the patient. Engaging in real dialogue with him or her will ensure full understanding, and minimise the resentment which may result in serious dissatisfaction, and, in some cases, litigation. In addition, the surgeon would do well to make use of other therapeutic professionals in facilitating the psychological and social rehabilitation which follows the surgical procedure. Help should be given to adapt to the changed body image which is the likely outcome of surgery, and to the consequent changed social roles. A plea is made for open communication between surgeon and patient, to ensure that realistic social goals are established.

The author showed in her original study (described above) that complaints amongst patients with slight disfigurement could be due to psychological difficulties unrelated to the defect. This is no excuse for poor surgery, but it does explain dissatisfaction with good surgery, and it is avoidable.

> ... if time were taken to look beyond the external deformity and to consider each patient as a total and unique personality and what significance the deformity has for him.[55]

She stresses the need for the surgeon to use professionals from other disciplines to assist in screening and counselling - psychiatrists, psychologists and social workers. However, she insists that these professionals, whose training traditionally has focused on a personal pathology of the behaviour of the individual, should see the disfigured person in the social context in which he or she lives:

> Such interpretations fail to consider the person in the context of his social, cultural and religious background, the influence of the social world in which he lives, and the impact of these factors on his attitudes and behaviour.[56]

She then provides two illustrations of failure by surgeons to recognise features of cases presented to them as coming from non-American cultures - the need for a Puerto Rican woman to have a scar removed, because it suggested that she had been unfaithful, and an Eastern European Jewish woman, who was deemed to be hostile to her daughter because of the ritual slapping which was part of her cultural norm. These are further illustrations of the danger of not viewing phenomena within their complete context.

## Success

A constant theme throughout Frances Macgegor's writing is the need to elicit the patient's view of success, rather than the surgeon's, particularly if the latter's is predominantly a functional one. Successful outcome of surgery is not about the surgeon's skill, but about how the patient views the defect.[57]

## The significance for surgeons of minor blemishes

In "Social and Psychological Considerations," in 1973,[58] the focus is on the assessment of patients for surgery. Professor Macgregor draws attention to the pitfalls which plastic surgeons face, and suggests why they may occur. In particular, she highlights the special difficulties posed by those with apparently minor disfigurements. In contrast to those with substantial disfigurement, which is evident and incontrovertible, those with scarcely perceptible disorders require further scrutiny, to consider their motivation for applying for surgery, and to see how large the disfigurement seems to them.

Excessive pre-occupation with a minor or non-existent blemish may be an indicator of neurosis, or a sign that the individual is pre-disposed to psychosis. Neither would exclude the patient automatically from surgery, but a psychiatric opinion would be indicated. Macgregor gives an illustration of a woman who underwent several episodes of cosmetic surgery, and who was still not satisfied with her appearance. More detailed investigation at an earlier stage would have shown excessive preoccupation and dissatisfaction with her body, which was neurotic in origin; the woman subsequently attempted suicide.

Overall, Macgregor found that:

- Those with minimal defects are 'inordinately concerned with and about themselves;
- Those with mild facial deviations have a more distorted body image than those who are severely impaired;
- Post-operatively, they tend to focus on minor imperfections.[59]

## Unrealistic expectations

Those with unrealistic social expectations of surgery are most likely to retaliate against the surgeon, and are likely to degenerate psychologically after surgery, since to operate on someone who is placing undue weight for their ills on the defect is to reinforce this belief, which cannot be fulfilled.

## The stresses of surgery itself

The process of seeking relief through surgery is stressful in itself. Surgeons need to be aware of the demoralising effect of long-term multi-stage rehabilitation, producing "rage, frustration and discouragement." In the case of those who rely in the sort term or longer term on prosthetic rehabilitation, there is also the fear of discovery, for example, if the prosthesis falls or moves out of place.[60]

In the process of rehabilitation, the patient must be helped to accept residual disfigurement. The pace of helping him or her to face such facts must be based on an appraisal of the individual, the need to keep hope going should be balanced with honesty, and the surgeon must not avoid this because of his or her own fear of the pain involved.[61]

In order to avoid pitfalls such as unrealistic expectations of surgery and motivation for surgery external to the patient, Macgregor advises that each patient should be counselled, and offers a checklist of features, any of which is cause to hold back plans for surgery, or to refer to a psychiatrist. They are largely the same as those referred to in Macgregor and Schaffner above, with one addition, "the wish to eliminate a feature similar to a rejected or rejecting parent".[62]

## Patients with a history of mental illness

Most surgeons, according to the author, try to avoid carrying out surgery on those with a known psychiatric history. This may not be fair to the individual:

> Most plastic surgeons have rules of thumb for deciding that a person is a risky candidate psychologically. Strict adherence to these rules, however, can preclude objective judgement, thereby depriving some people of the attention they deserve.[63]

Nonetheless, the fact remains that surgeons need guidelines, and so do regard psychiatric treatment as a lasting indicator that they should not proceed with surgery.

Plastic surgeons have one of the highest records for suits of malpractice, and so surgeons are cautious about operating on a patient whom they feel would be vindictive if the results were not good. In practice this may deny patients access to treatment, on the basis of past events and present suspicion.

## Lawyers

The fact that a lawyer is involved in a matter of facial reconstruction means that the relationship between patient and surgeon has broken down. The emphasis of the message to lawyers is two-fold: first, she explains why patients set so much store by the positive or negative outcome of surgery, and second, she explains how the doctor may have contributed to the breakdown.

In "Traumatic facial injuries and the law" in 1973,[64] a range of empirical studies is drawn on in order to demonstrate that:

> ... not only does an unsightly face impede a person's chances for a normal and productive life but ... the social, psychological and economic consequences may be even more grave than those resulting from damage to other parts of the body.[65]

She draws attention to the significance of the face for social intercourse, as a means of communicating a range of fine thoughts, feelings and personality traits. Disfigurement reduces the impact of the face as a means of showing the self to others, and causes the individual to retire from social life far more completely than other disabilities necessarily do. There is a felt shame, because of the loss of such a significant part of the self. This is exacerbated by our heavy emphasis on physical beauty. The amount of loss and shame experienced is not necessarily related to the extent of disfigurement; this has been demonstrated in several studies by Frances Macgregor.

Two major economic consequences of disfigurement are named: first, in the short to medium term, illness and reconstructive surgery is extensive, and disruptive to lives; it is virtually impossible to be able to predict that one is going to be well enough to sustain a job, to be there, and to be a full participant at work.

Secondly, the earning power of the person who is facially disfigured is less than that of other people; employers are unwilling to hire those whose appearance is not pleasing to colleagues, customers and members of the public. Several illustrations are given of this, and also cites a report by the New York State Employment Service, which shows that:

> ... three-fourths of the job placements for disfigured persons were made in unskilled occupations, jobs that were 'behind the scenes,' where the person would not be seen by the public.[66]

By means of two case illustrations,[67] it is argued that the psychological and even economic cost of traumatic facial injury is potentially as much as that of functional impairment, and should be considered in lawsuits for compensation. The author describes the significance of the face for social existence, and as a contributor to the quality of human life, and asserts that that quality is reduced as a consequence of facial injury.

This is not a research article; it is a set of precepts for trial lawyers, based on research findings which are reported elsewhere, an application of academic work to a professional situation.

The third of Frances Macgregor's articles on the law and plastic surgery[68] looks at the origins of litigation within the surgeon's own handling of the case. She asks why medical litigation is on the increase, and in particular why the plastic surgeon is so vulnerable. It may well be that the general emphasis on youth, appearance and self-gratification has caused greater reliance to be placed on plastic surgery. Accompanying this has been an increasing emphasis on gaining one's rights, and a seeking of redress when they are infringed.

One of the principal causes of litigation is the failure of the surgeon to communicate adequately with the patient:

> An analysis of the difficulties and conflicts that emerge between doctors and patients will show that many are not solely the consequence of unfulfilled expectations or poor surgical results, but have their roots in or are exacerbated by the quality of interaction between doctor and patient and the attitudes and behaviour of the surgeon in the course of the relationship".[69]

In addition to Professor Macgregor's own research over the years, she cites the views of a trial attorney:

'Doctors are their own worst enemies,' contends an attorney whose speciality is medical litigation. 'I tell them over and over, if only they would take a little more time, have a little more feeling, they wouldn't be subject to lawsuits.'[70]

A study is referred to in which physicians were asked whether certain patients were suit-prone. Those who did not feel the threat of litigation were those who spoke of a relationship with the patient.

If a surgeon minimises the patients' complaints, resentment will ensue. It is acknowledged that the surgeon's priority must be to spend time in theatre; this makes any time he or she spends with the patient most valued, and studies suggest that the investment is worthwhile. The time spent must involve two-way communication, rather than the straight imparting by the surgeon of facts.

The very image of plastic surgery is provocative. Advertising for plastic surgery presents it as easy, attractive, and achieving excellent results very quickly. It is also very costly, and there are examples of surgeons who have clearly benefitted from a lucrative practice. This may stimulate the dissatisfied patient to feel that the surgeon has literally benefitted at his or her expense. Such excesses are hard to control.


**Social workers**

Although all of Frances Macgregor's work stresses the importance of social factors far more than psychological ones, she has written little to link her research directly with social work. It can be argued that all of it is applicable, but in few cases does she make the last link by helping social practitioners in the day-to-day content of their work. She is not a social worker, and this could well be the reason for her failure to propose a model of intervention.

One article relating to social work with children with ear defects has already been mentioned.[71] In a further article addressed to social workers in 1980,[72] awareness is raised of the problems which may face congenitally disfigured children in general and their families. It provides insights, giving case illustrations, although it is not intended to suggest detailed techniques of intervention.

The greatest problem for the child either born with or acquiring a disfigurement is likely to be the social environment, which is likely to be hostile, curious and ridiculing:

From the time a child with a facial anomaly enters school, if not before, he will discover that, even though he is capable of doing what other children do, he is an object of curiosity or pity, that he may be the butt of cruel jokes, nicknames and teasing, that his privacy is invaded by staring and questions, and that he will attract few, if any, friends.[73]

There is a need for the parents of such a child to be helped in many ways by professionals and friends, but particularly by them being open and straightforward, from the very beginning - telling them of the full extent of the condition, and the realistic outcomes of corrective surgery. The parents themselves must begin by acknowledging fully the disfigurement, and offering the same warm acceptance which any child needs to grow up with a healthy, normal personality. They can only do this by first recognising the difficulty which they face in doing so.

The role of the social worker is emphasised, as a listener, as a link between the family and the clinical team, and between the home and school, when the child begins his or her education.

These insights are derived from Professor Macgregor's research experience - she makes extensive use of well-selected case illustrations in this article, which is addressed to social workers. It is not establishing a theoretical framework for intervention - Macgregor is not a social worker - she is an anthropologist and sociologist - but it highlights issues and areas of concern to which social workers must give attention, just as elsewhere she offers insights to other professionals, for example orthodontists and lawyers.

**Conclusion**

1. For more than forty years, Frances Macgregor has studied the social context of those with facial deformity or disfigurement - considering what is normal, what is abnormal, and what can be done about facial deformity, including the place of plastic surgery, and an evaluation of its effectiveness.

2. The significance of the face is emphasised, first as a means of communication, and second as a social asset within a society dominated by aspirations to approximate to the norm of beauty. Whether or not the individual aspires to fit into this expectation, the disfigured person suffers a significant primary

disadvantage by not being able to communicate effectively: speech itself may be impaired, eating as a social medium is restricted, but most of all the visible differentness of disfigurement denies the disfigured person automatic access to normal social intercourse.

3. Those who seek surgery are described - particularly those with a congenital deformity or differentness. Generally, they are not vain people, but rather they wish to be assimilated into society without any of the self-consciousness or emotional pain which being different causes. There are some exceptions, and those whose expectations of the social benefits of surgery are unrealistic should be counselled away from such a course. Generally, what makes people happy with the outcome of surgery is not the technical standard of the work so much as the attitude of the surgeon, and the realism of the patient's own attitude to the operation.

4. When the individual undergoes surgery in order to improve a facial deformity, he or she must be helped to understand that plastic surgery is not a perfect solution; there is almost sure to be a residual disfigurement. The first step towards getting the patient to accept this is for the surgeon to accept it; this is not always easy, but if he or she fails to accept it, the patient is not going to be convinced.

5. Professor Macgregor describes in detail the impact of deformity on the life of the individual. She says, for example, that impact on family life is most pronounced when it is a child who is disfigured. She refers to a range of strategies adopted in order to survive, many of them very similar to Goffman's typology - denial, self-conscious preparedness, withdrawal and seclusion, aggression, blaming others, avoidance, and using the deformity as a defence or justification of other shortcomings.

6. A number of lessons and precepts are offered to professionals dealing with disfigured people, particularly surgeons but also lawyers and social workers. In particular, the absolute need for openness is stressed, for good communication, and for a trusting relationship between surgeon and patient.

7. Much of Frances Macgregor's experience was of congenital

deformity- certainly this was the main focus of her empirical work. The present empirical study will consider how far her experience may be applied to those who require surgery for the treatment of cancer. For example, in the latter case, are there any social indicators for not proceeding with surgery? It may well be that in the case of cancer patients the need to act quickly and operate supersedes every other consideration, but where, unlike in Macgregor's experience, a range of therapies is possible, social factors may be influential in determining the preferred treatment.


**Notes**

1.  Macgregor, F.C., 'Social and psychological studies of plastic surgery', in *Clinics in Plastic Surgery*, 9, 3, pp. 283-288, 198.
2.  op. cit., p. 284.
3.  op. cit., p. 285.
4.  Macgregor, F.C., 1979. *After Plastic Surgery (Adaptation and Adjustment)*, J.F. Bergin, New York.
5.  Macgregor, F.C. and Schaffner, B., 1950, 'Screening patients for nasal plastic operations' *Psychomatic Medicine*, 12, 5, pp. 277-291, September/October.
6.  Details of Macgregor's sample are confusing: one forms the impression of a rolling programme of research over many years, with patients overlapping from one study or publication to another. In 1950, Macgregor refers to a sample of 73 patients applying for rhinoplasty. Then in the following year she describes 115 patients seen over the same period, presumably including some or all of the nasal patients. In 1953 she referred to the "74 patients studied during the course of the Project" Then, in 1967, she describes 89 rhinoplasty patients collected between 1946 and 1954. Finally, in her follow-up study of 1979, she interviews 16 of the 71 patients previously studied, 20 years on. Nowhere is the sample the same, but how much overlap there is is most unclear - 73, 115, 74, 89, and 71.
7..  Macgregor, F.C., Abel, T.M., Bryt, A., Laner, E., and Weissmann, S.; 1953, *Facial Deformities and Plastic Surgery: a Psychosocial Study*, Charles C. Thomas, Springfield, Ill.
8.  op. cit., p. 89.
9.  op. cit., p. 95.
10. op. cit., p. 100.

11. Macgregor, F.C., 1951, 'Some psycho-social problems associated with facial deformities', *American Sociological Review*, 16, 5, pp. 629-638,October.

12. Macgregor, F.C., 1967, 'Social and cultural components in themotivations of persons seeking plastic surgery of the nose', *Journal of Health and Social Behaviour*, 8, 2.

13. op. cit., p. 129.

14. op. cit., p. 140.

15. Macgregor, F.C., 1979, *After Plastic Surgery (Adaptation and Adjustment)*, J.F. Bergin, New York.

16. op. cit., p. 106.

17. op. cit., p. 107.

18. ibid.

19. op. cit., p. 111.

20. op. cit., p. 116.

21. op. cit., p. 630.

22. op. cit., p. 632.

23. 1953, op. cit., p. 70.

24. op. cit., p. 76.

25. op. cit., p. 77.

26. Macgregor, F.C., 1974, *Transformation and Identity - The Face and Plastic Surgery*, Quadrangle/The New York Times Book Company, New York.

27. op. cit., p. 30.

28. op. cit., p. 60.

29. Macgregor, F.C., 1970, 'Social and psychological implications of dento-facial disfigurement', *The Angle Orthodontist*, 40, 3, pp. 231-233.

30. op. cit., p. 233, from Goffman, E., 1963, *Encounters: Two Studies in the Sociology of Interaction*, Bobbs-Merrill Co., Indianapolis.

31. 1953, op. cit., p. 63.

32. ibid.

33. 1951, op. cit., p. 632.

34. 1951, op. cit.

35. Macgregor, F.C., 1978, 'Ear deformities: social and psychological implications', *Clinics in Plastic Surgery*, 5, 3, July.

36. 1953, op. cit., p. 65.

37. 1974, op. cit., pp. 34-5.

38. 1953, op. cit.

39. 1953, op. cit.

40. op. cit., p.83.
41. discussed again in 1974, op. cit.
42. Macgregor, F.C., and Ford, B., 1971, 'The other face of plastic surgery: the disappointed patient', *Science Digest*, pp. 16-20, April.
43. op. cit., p. 20.
44. Macgregor, F.C., 1981, 'Patient dissatisfaction with results of technically satisfactory surgery', *Aesthetic Plastic Surgery*, pp. 27-32.
45. Macgregor, F.C., 1953, 'Some psychological hazards of plastic surgery of the face', *Plastic and Reconstructive Surgery*, 12, 2, Based on a lecture given at the American Academy of Opthalmology and Otolaryngology, Chicago, 1951.
46. op. cit., p. 124.
47. 1982, op. cit., p. 391.
48. 1974, op. cit., p. 444.
49. 1974, op. cit., p. 446.
50. Macgregor, F.C., 1982, 'Surgery: the patient and the surgeon', *Clinics in Plastic Surgery*, 9, 3, pp. 387-395, July.
51. op. cit., p. 389.
52. Macgregor, F.C., 'Social and Psychological Considerations', Chapter 3 in Rees, T.D. and Wood-Smith, D., 1973, *Cosmetic Facial Surgery*, W.B. Saunders, Philadelphia, p. 31.
53. Macgregor, F.C., 1976, 'Aesthetic plastic surgery: some caveats', *Aesthetic Plastic Surgery*, 1, 1 pp. 71-80.
54. op. cit., p. 72.
55. 1951, op. cit., p. 125.
56. 1973, op. cit., p. 32.
57. 1974, op. cit.
58. 1973, op. cit.
59. 1976, op. cit.
60. 1974, op. cit.
61. ibid.
62. 1951, op. cit., p. 129.
63. 1973, op. cit., p. 29.
64. Macgregor, F.C., 1973. 'Traumatic facial injuries and the law: some social, psychological and economic ramifications', *Trial Lawyers Quarterly*, Vol. 9, 4, Fall, pp.50-53.
65. op. cit., p. 51.
66. op. cit., p. 53.
67. Macgregor, F.C., 1984, 'Psychic trauma of facial disfigurement', *Trial*, January.

68. Macgregor, F.C., 1984, 'Cosmetic surgery: a sociological analysis of litigation and a surgical speciality', *Aesthetic Plastic Surgery*, 8, p. 219-224.
69. op. cit., p. 220.
70. ibid.
71. 1978, op. cit.
72. Macgregor, F.C., 1980, 'The facially disfigured child', *Pediatric Social Work*, 1, 1.
73. op. cit., p. 1.

# 3 Professional perspectives

This chapter represents the views of a range of practical people - either professionals such as surgeons, psychologists, psychiatrists and social workers, or those who have conducted field research only - predominantly psychologists.

First, the professional orientation of the authors is considered, and how this influences their contributions. Next, the theoretical assumptions and values of the writers is described - particularly in relation to the significance of the face. Third, the empirical works are reviewed, and a profile provided of the patients who are studied. Outcomes of surgery follow, positive and negative, and views described on what contributes to positive outcomes. Fifth, aspects and features which contribute to survival and successful rehabilitation are described, and finally, practical advice on how to help patients in this process is summarised.

## Professional orientation

The professional disciplines represented are numerous; hence the principal focus of the papers is widely varied. It is important to understand the professional stance of each author or authors, as one part of an evaluation of their contribution to the discussion. This section summarises this contribution by considering the following aspects of each paper:

1.  The profession or professions represented;
2.  Whether the paper has a theoretical or empirical basis;
3.  How the professional standpoint helps in the understanding of disfigurement;
4.  How the profession contributes to rehabilitation.

All but one group are providers of services. The exception is the group of experimental psychologists from North East London Polytechnic, Ray Bull and others. Of the five papers contributed by this group, four are field studies, and one is a survey of literature. In the empirical papers, the results of controlled studies are described, not of disfigured people, but of those who react to apparent disfigurement. Their work follows strict experimental rules, and the results help us to see the impact which the face makes on everyday social transactions, such as meeting in the street, or helping other individuals. There is little reference to rehabilitation of or help for disfigured people, although the authors do assert that their work may contribute to these areas.

The principal research papers with a psychiatric basis within the studies described originate from the Hospital for Sick Children in Toronto. They also represent a strongly collaborative element, involving a range of disciplines. Table 3.1 summarises the professions who wrote these papers, and the broad theme of each paper, illustrating the contribution which each profession can make to issues of deformity and disfigurement.

**Table 3.1**
**Summary of Toronto Papers**

| Author | Date | Profession(s) | | | | | Comment |
|---|---|---|---|---|---|---|---|
| | | Social Worker | Psycho metrist | Plastic Surgeon | Psych iatry | Psyc holog y | |
| Munro | 1975 | | | * | | | Importance of team work |
| Lefebvre | 1978 | | | * | * | | satisfaction with surgery and its psychological impact |
| Lefebvre & Barclay | 1982 | * | | | * | | psychosocial improvement after surgery |
| Arndt et al. (1) | 1986 | * | * | * | * | * | improved appearance, self-esteem and social performance |
| Arndt & al. (2) | 1986 | * | * | * | * | | psychosocial consequences of surgery |

All but the first by Ian Munro, a Scottish plastic surgeon, are empirical works. His strongly expressed plea for collaboration between the disciplines was based upon his experience as a plastic surgeon. The subsequent four papers describing empirical research are all collaborative, and all but one involve Ian Munro himself. The common author to all these four is Arlette Lefebvre, a child psychiatrist, and the studies are structured and reported very much in the tradition of clinical psychology, involving the use of scales to rate performance and satisfaction. These collaborative works are concerned almost exclusively with children.

The next group of authors consists of those who have conducted empirical studies of head and neck cancer, its social or psychological consequences, its treatment and rehabilitation. Eight studies are referred to, and these are summarised in Table 3.2.

### Table 3.2
### Empirical Studies of Patients with Head and Neck Cancer

| Author | Date | Profession(s) | | | | Comment |
|--------|------|----------------|------|------|------|---------|
| | | Social Worker | Biolo gist | Type of Surgeon | Psycho logist | |
| Rozen & al. | 1972 | * | * | Dental | | Social and psychological functioning after treatment. Management of problems and rehabilitation |
| West | 1973 | | | | * | How people adapt and get on with others following surgery |
| Sela & Lowental | 1980 | | | Oral | | Self-image, optimism and feeling of health after prosthetic rehabilitation |
| Fiegenbaum | 1981 | | | | * | Social training to raise self-confidence and reduce anxiety after surgery |
| David & Barritt | 1982 | * | | Plastic | | Psychological measures of quality of life in treated head and neck cancer. Rehabilitation. Management of dying patients |
| Morton & al. | 1984 | | | ENT | * | Psychological measures of quality of life in treated head and neck cancer patients |

'continued'

| Roefs & al. | 1984 | | | Oral and dental | * | Psychological factors affecting acceptance of facial prosthesis |
| Ildstad & al. | 1989 | | | General and plastic | | Age, stage of tumour and its location as determinants of survival |

But two of the studies involved surgeons. The exceptions are West, a research psychologist, and Fiegenbaum, a clinical psychologist, but both were based in practice settings. Two social workers feature - one in the article by Rozen et al.[1] all of whom are members of staff at the University of California Maxillo-facial Rehabilitation Clinic, where it is stressed that a team approach is used to facilitate the rehabilitation of cancer patients who require prosthetic work following treatment for facial cancer. The other is in the paper written by David and Barritt[2] -

J.A. Barritt is the social worker - and the influence of the social worker is evident in the features which are considered important when planning the rehabilitation of the person who has suffered from head or neck cancer:

- The social value of the face and mouth;
- Emotional responses to the diagnosis;
- Post-operative depression - this occurred for all patients, but was particularly severe for the ten patients for whom an endogenous element already existed;
- Body image - the fear of mutilation, and the subsequent need to acquire a new body image;
- Stresses and difficulties which illness and treatment present to the family;
- Adaptation - changed appearance following survival, dependency on the treatment centre. In South Australia, many patients live a long way from the treatment centre, and this provokes a fear of isolation from vital sources of help;
- Fear 'of death, and stages of becoming aware of the closeness of death;
- Controlling pain, and overcoming practical difficulties, including speaking, swallowing, and reducing offensive odours. All of these have emotional and social aspects to them, in addition to them being a practical issue.

The final study referred to in Table 3.3, Ildstad et al.[3] is important more for what it omits than what it says - it is a major study of survival - the possible determinants of survival were subjected to statistical analysis, and three variables were found to have significance -age of patient, site of tumour, and stage of tumour development when treatment was sought. Age was the only significant variable, but gender was also considered in the study, and found not to be significant. The study used a large data base, and could have been used to assist more in understanding the social determinants of ill-health.

A further two empirical studies included no head and neck cancer patients; these are summarised in Table 3.3.

### Table 3.3
### Other Empirical Studies

| Author | Date | Profession(s) | | | | Comment |
|--------|------|------|------|------|------|---------|
| | | Medical Student | Neurol ogist | Psych iatrist | Psycho logist | |
| Roback & al. | 1981 | * | * | * | | Communication skills training, individual case study |
| Kalick | 1982 | | | | * | Stresses the value of inter-disciplinary collaboration. Good theoretical base, particularly from social psychology and sociology |

Although a range of disciplines contributed to the paper written by Roback et al.[4] in fact the approach is broadly psychiatric, being a skills training programme for an individual person suffering from neurofibromatosis. The other of these two papers is written by Kalick[5] a psychologist, and he stresses the value of collaboration between disciplines, and is especially good at using written sociological material to inform multi-disciplinary practice.

The final group of papers is entirely theoretical, although informed by the practice experience of the contributors. Their contribution is summarised in Table 3.5, showing how the profession of the author influences the approach taken to a broadly similar issue. In one paper (Constable and Bernstein)[6], the profession(s) of the authors is not stated, but a psychological approach is taken.

## Table 3.4
## Theoretical Studies

| Author | Date | Profession(s) | | | | Comment |
|---|---|---|---|---|---|---|
| | | Social Worker | Type of Surgeon | Psychi atrist | Psycho logist | |
| Riley | 1968 | | Prosthod ontic | | | Predominantly technical aspects of rehabilitation, some brief references to sympathetic handling of patients |
| Peterson & Topazian | 1974 | | Oral | | | Checklist for screening patients, some emphasis placed on protection of surgeon |
| Addison | 1975 | * | | | | Social worker, drawing predominantly on psycho-social theory |
| Bailey & Edwards | 1975 | | | | * | Psychological issues associated with prosthetics, drawing together several strands of the literature |
| Frank | 1975 | | | * | | Psychiatrist addressing prosthetic technicians on their counselling role |
| Light | 1976 | | Dental | | | Need for surgeon to be aware of psychological factors |
| Constables & Bernstein | 1979 | not known | | | | The psychology of reactions to disfigurement |
| Nordlicht | 1979 | | | * | | Psychopathology of facial disfigurement |
| Stricker | 1979 | Dental research staff, large psychological component | | | | A thorough drawing together of several theoretical strands |
| Van Doorne | 1981 | | Prosthod ontic | | | Surgeon, talking to technicians, about psychology of disfigurement |

Four of the authors are surgeons, and three are addressing issues of concern to surgeons. The exception is Van Doorne[7] who is addressing maxillo-facial technicians about their role in the rehabilitative process. He summarises the literature on the rehabilitation of head and neck cancer patients, suggesting that more needs to be done to discover what makes a prosthesis acceptable. Work already carried out suggests that prostheses which facilitate eating and speaking are accepted more readily than those which are extra-oral, and only cosmetic.

Of the remaining three surgeons, Riley is concerned mostly with the technical aspects of prosthetic work; Light gives a useful short paper on psychological factors which surgeons need to be aware of; the most substantial contribution is made by Peterson and Topazian of the Medical College of Georgia.[8] The authors, both oral surgeons, have produced a format for the pre-operative interview, to ensure that all relevant fields of information are covered, and to provide an outline for the writing up of the report. Although the typology may be of use to professionals other than oral surgeons, there is an assumption made that the oral surgeon alone will carry out the assessment (with a psychiatrist in some instances), and there is little reference to the team approach described elsewhere in the literature.

The objective of orthognathic surgery is defined as patient happiness, and it is accepted that surgical skill is not always the determinant of patient satisfaction:

> Post-operative dissatisfaction is not necessarily related to the surgical skill of the surgeon, but results primarily from mutual failure of communication between the surgeon and the patient.[9]

Unfortunately, Peterson and Topazian stress the negative consequences of such dissatisfaction to the surgeon (complaints, non-payment of fee, litigation) more than the impact on the patient. However, this does not invalidate their checklist, and the observations which they make on each point. The areas of evaluation are as follows:

1. Degree of facial deformity;
2. Duration of patient concern;
3. Nature of deformity - acquired (how long ago) or developmental;
4. State of social adjustment;
5. Role of deformity in current personality;
6. Source of motivation;
7. Expectations from surgery.

It will be noted that all seven issues are social rather than surgical. It is regrettable that a team approach was not considered by Peterson and Topazian; particularly when social judgements are being made (such as the level of a person's stability), the opinions of other professionals would have provided invaluable insights. Nonetheless, the interview schedule has a useful content, and systematises what otherwise might be a completely subjective decision.

There is one social worker in this group, Addison[10], who was also addressing an audience of maxillo-facial technicians. She was speaking at the same conference as was Franks[11], a psychiatrist, whose paper is also considered here. Franks, a consultant psychiatrist at Queen Mary Hospital, Roehampton, stresses the value to the patient of a caring and positive attitude on the part of the maxillo-facial technician, who actually constructs the prosthesis for a patient who loses facial tissue due to cancer:

> Because of the close contact between the technician and the patient during a critical phase of rehabilitation, he has a major part to play in the management of the psychological and social problems associated with this. If he is able to build a warm and understanding relationship with the patient he will then be in a position to greatly help the patient in what will be a very difficult time.[12]

Frank offers advice to the technician on how to empathise with the withdrawn patient, enabling him or her to express painful feelings. The technician is in a good position to do so, "... since he is seen as being a person who provides practical help in the problems of re-adjustment." The practice experience on which Frank draws is no doubt substantial, but the paper says nothing new, and also appears to talk down to the maxillo-facial technician; the latter is counselled that he or she is not a psychological expert, although still be of use to the patient:

> ... if he reinforces the empathy and understanding of an intelligent layman with experience and a little knowledge, he will be highly effective ...[13]

The remainder of the contributors are psychologists and one psychiatrist, Nordlicht[14], who offers a pathological viewpoint of the patient's ability to recover successfully. Much the same issue was encountered in Macgregor's work, when the initial predictions of failure of patients to be rehabilitated did not materialise. Nordlicht assumes the possibility of psychopathology in every instance.

## The importance of the face

Ray Bull and his associates, of North East London Polytechnic, are experimental psychologists, and in the course of the 1980s they considered the effect of appearance on human behaviour. They looked at the impact of appearance on the willingness of people to help, on criminality, and at a range of attitudes and behaviours of children and adults in relation to disfigured people.

Bull and Stevens[15] referred to the literature on the effect of appearance on people's preparedness to help others. They found that it was inconclusive and contradictory. Their own field experiment was carried out to learn whether disfigured people were justified in their assertion that their disfigurement discouraged people from helping them.

Their study took the form of a house-to-house collection for a recognised children's charity. At half the houses visited, the collector was made up as if she had a facial port-wine stain. Two other variables were employed - half of the collections were made from high rise flats, and half from middle class semi-detached houses, and in half the occasions the collector held the gaze of the donor (in order to induce a greater rapport). Donors consistently gave more, and there were fewer refusals, when the collector did not have the stain.

The results appeared to support the hypothesis that disfigured people are disadvantaged in seeking help. However, this was a contrived experiment, and how transferable it is to every day behaviour is open to question. Furthermore, the ethics of provoking more or less generous behaviour in unsuspecting individuals, who believed that they were simply giving (or not) to charity, may also be challenged.

However, such social disadvantage was not found in a further study by the same authors[16], who found no evidence that facially attractive people acquire greater conversational expertise than those who are judged not so attractive.

In the course of their study of the problems encountered by disfigured people, Rumsey et al. (essentially the same research group) conducted a field experiment[17] to see whether observed members of the public would stand as close to a disfigured person as to a person without disfigurement. Someone with a made-up port-wine stain stood at a pedestrian crossing, during a busy lunch hour period. It was found that people stood on the non-disfigured side of the confederate many times more frequently than on the disfigured side.

Rumsey et al.'s study is conducted with the highest rigour, and the results were most significant. Nonetheless they are not convincing when they attempt to relate their contrived observation to everyday circumstances. The generalisation made by way of introduction to ".... increasing numbers of road accidents, industrial injuries, muggings, and terrorist bombings"[18] is matched in the conclusion when the results are interpreted by saying that ".... people are generally sympathetic, but are unsure how to behave when confronted with a novel stimulus in the shape of a facial disfigurement." They further justify more study because of ".... the long National Health Service waiting lists in Britain for the revision of facial disfigurements" and suggest that their findings could be used to ".... facilitate the teaching of social skills to the disfigured."[19]

None of these suggestions, interpretations or justifications is substantiated, in contrast to the rigour of the study itself.

Rumsey et al. reinforced the findings of this study in a further experiment[20], in which older children (around eleven years) associated the faces of adults who had minor disfigurements with negative feelings, and ascribed positive feelings to the same adults when their disfigurements had been corrected by surgery.

Bull[21] reviewed studies of the assumed association between facial deformity and criminality, and found that a highly significant link existed between the two. Members of the public are able, more often than not, to identify which members of a group of people were the perpetrators of crime, and even to identify the crime with which individuals are associated, based on appearance alone. He also reported on several experimental programmes of plastic surgery within the American prison service, in which the recidivism of those who underwent corrective facial surgery was significantly reduced.

It is not possible to conclude from these studies that behaviour can be predicted universally by examining facial appearance. Nor can it be said that behaviour can always be adapted merely by adapting appearance. Bull does not go as far as to say that appearance causes criminality, but he expresses an interest in determining whether a causative link does exist. In the process, he does not raise the possibility that these two factors, rather than having a causative link, might be caused by a third variable. This might be at least as plausible.

The research of Bull and his associates does show that members of the public (strangers) place a negative value on facial disfigurement in a number of practical ways - they are less generous to facially disfigured people, they distance themselves spatially from them, and they make assumptions that they possess negative behavioural attributes. Macgregor's work has provided many illustrations of the fact that disfigured people are aware of such ratings, and have adopted a range of strategies to manage the discomfort. Some of these strategies will be described later in this chapter.

Speaking at an international prosthetics workshop, Carol Addison[22], a social worker based at the time at Queen Mary's Hospital, Roehampton, referred to the practical problems which the person with a facial prosthesis encounters, but emphasises that the disfigurement is more a social handicap than a physical one, since the individual without normal appearance is seen as not quite human. Physical attractiveness is seen as necessary in order to achieve success in career and personal relationships, since it is used as an indicator of personality and intelligence. This is all the more so if the disfigurement has reduced expressive ability, as it usually does in some way.

The American plastic surgeons Constable and Bernstein[23] also attempted some explanation of these phenomena, referring to the limited tolerance by the public of unsightly people, for which they cited a range of explanations:

- The damaged individual frightens the person who is whole;[24]
- The face is not hidden, and is always a reminder of the shortcoming;
- The sense organs are contained within the face. There is a tendency to greater aversion if communication with the disfigured person is also reduced, for example by speech impairment;
- The face is the means of recognition;
- Good looks are seen to make us more valuable, because of society's quest for beauty.

Because professionals tend to maintain intellectual control over their feelings, they may not exhibit all of these reactions, but doctors should be aware of an additional feeling which they may have about facial disfigurement, especially as a residue of surgery, namely their dislike of chronic illness and disability, as it is not susceptible to improvement by their skills.

Bailey and Edwards[25] (who are prosthetic dental surgeons based in San Diego, California) emphasised the role of the body as a medium for communicating with the world through all the senses. The outcome of these communication experiences contributes to body image. The individual is therefore highly dependent on those parts of the body which aid communication:

> To the extent that a particular part of the body aids in receiving or expressing information, the person loves and needs that organ. Alteration, impairment, or loss of that part involves emotional turmoil. A strong sense of despair and depression typically accompanies the impairment or loss of a body part.[26]

In particular, the face is of importance, as from earliest infancy, it assists the individual to establish full communication with the world. Its importance is illustrated and further enhanced by the value placed on attractiveness. The authors observe that "the cosmetic industries experience staggering profits from the concern most people have for the beauty of the maxillo-facial region."[27] This is only one side of the story - to a large extent it is the cosmetic industries which stimulate the concern for beauty of the face. Throughout life facial importance is substantial - the social nature of communal meals, and the expression of intimacy, are two situations in which the face plays a part.

When part of the face is lost, part of the self is lost, and psychological impairment may occur. A whole range of new experiences must be gone through - wondering how others will react, getting used to new sensory experiences, acceptance of the new body shape, possible reduced social status.

However, those with the greatest disfigurement do not always experience the most distress. Bailey and Edwards suggest that

> ...the patient's self-perceptions, emotional stability, personality characteristics, and social circumstances appear to be the salient factors in dealing with maxillo-facial disorders and the rehabilitation process.[28]

For this reason, the need for a good surgeon/patient relationship is stressed; there is no substitute for clear communication.

This theme was further developed by Stricker et al.,[29] at the U.S. National Institute of Dental Research. The self-image of a disfigured individual derives, not from the disfigurement itself, but from societal attachment of stigma to those who are different, the definition of difference being defined and constantly redefined by society. Freud's emphasis on the body experience as the core of personality has been developed and enhanced. The "self" has become associated with the body, and its specific parts, particularly the chest. Consequently, one may anticipate that physical deformity will mark a threat to the self:

> Many of the most troublesome reactions to body damage are not due to damage, per se, but to the meaning of body damage in the total life structure of the individual.[30]

Similarly, improvement in body structure does not necessarily produce enhanced mood or functioning. Depression may follow a favourable improvement to the body, because of unrealistic expectations of improvement to the personality, or because of an unfavourable reaction to loss, no matter how unwanted was the thing that was lost.

> ... the person loses something around which his whole personality structure may well have been built. He loses hope that physical changes will produce psychological improvement. With that hope gone, as much of the personality structure will collapse as was initially dependent upon that expectation.[31]

Stricker et al. consider the effects of disfigurement on interpersonal relationships, stating that malformation affects attractiveness, which in turn affects the making of relationships. Their survey of other studies concludes that deviations from the normal are not negatively rated unless they are extreme deviations. Studies vary on the matter of the relative importance of different attributes (some attributes or facial expressions have a potentially complex interpretation, and therefore may be misinterpreted), but in almost every study the extent to which the chin protrudes or recedes is considered significant; the teeth are also considered to be a salient attribute - correctly aligned teeth are associated with sincerity, intelligence and conscientiousness.

To some extent society determines the norm of what is beautiful. Anthropological studies tell us that in some societies mutilations (such as those of the teeth) are highly esteemed, to the extent that the person who has not mutilated himself or herself is an outsider. Those who do not approximate to this societal norm must develop strategies of compensation, but this is difficult, because there is no one consistent societal response to deformity. The authors refer to the difficulties experienced by unattractive children in interaction with their peers, and note that they also exhibit more disturbed behaviour. Possibly this role is imposed on them because of the unpopularity induced by their appearance:

... the more minor physical anomalies young physical children have (for example, abnormal head circumference, epicanthal folds, widely spaced eyes, and curved fifth finger), the more aggressive, impulsive, or withdrawn behaviours they display, the less peer interaction they show, and the more negatively they are judged by their peers.[32]

Beauty is a highly prized component of desirability in adult relationships, probably the paramount component. Stricker et al. refer to the SVR (Stimulus-Value-Role) theory of interpersonal relationships, in which a three-stage process occurs during the selection of marital partners. The theory's relevance to this discussion is that the predominant stimulus towards intimacy is a visual one, and people with a facial deformity do not even achieve sufficiency in many people's opinion in the early stages of the making of a relationship.

Self-esteem and self-image are not objective realities; they change from person to person, and the rating of an individual alters depending on whether one is listening to the self-appraisal of the affected person, of someone close to him, or that of a total stranger. Lefebvre (a consultant child psychiatrist) and Barclay (a social worker) conducted a major study[33] of 250 children and adults aged six weeks to 39 years who attended the Hospital for Sick Children in Toronto. There was strong evidence that the image which patients had of themselves differed from that held by others. On the whole, Lefebvre and Barclay found that a person with a facial deformity rates it as less severe than do those around him, such as his parents (Mothers are slightly more severe than fathers in their ratings). The only notable exception is in the instance of adolescents, who tend to rate their deformities as at least as severe as others do. This was also found in Macgregor's studies. Congenitally disfigured patients see themselves as severely disfigured, as do oncology patients.

It is important to remember, when referring to disfigurement, that much of it will have been caused by therapeutic intervention - particularly for the eradication of cancer. Riley,[34] an American prosthodontic surgeon, fully acknowledges the psychological impact on the patient of the loss of tissue through cancer:

> The loss of an ear, nose, eye, or parts of the palate presents a psychologic, functional, and aesthetic burden that is difficult for the average individual to accept. It is also an economic and sociologic crisis if the deformity precludes the patient's gainful employment.[35]

The lesson so far established is that disfigured people are socially disadvantaged, particularly at the point of first encounter. This is due to the importance of the face in enabling clear communication to take place. The loss or disfigurement of part of the face results in a social hurt far more than a physical one. Such loss will be felt particularly keenly at certain times in the individual's life cycle.

## Profile of patients

Within the thirty papers reviewed in this chapter a substantial range of views is expressed, the product of professional experience, reviews of others' work, and direct empirical work carried out by the authors themselves. More than half of the papers reflect the results of first-hand empirical work, and it is important to note who exactly comprise the samples referred to, and what their characteristics are.

It is clear from Table 3.1 which works are empirical, and which are more general or theoretical. This section expands the empirical or theoretical base in more detail, by describing the principal focus of each author, and where the social and clinical characteristics of the groups of patients are described, a summary is provided.

Seventeen of the papers describe empirical studies, but five of them are distinctly different from the rest: these are the studies carried out at North-West London Polytechnic by Bull and his associates. The difference is two-fold: first, generally the disfigured person or persons are not really so; they are people without disfigurement made up to appear deformed or disfigured, or they are photographs of people without a recognisable deformity, introduced for the purposes of the experiment. Second, the people who are being studied are not those with the disfigurement, real or otherwise, but those who react to them, passers-by in the street, or people who open doors to charity collectors. So the samples are not samples in the accepted sense - they are not a carefully selected group of people with certain facial characteristics, but rather a range of members of the public who are assumed to represent average attitudes; the experimenters simply kept going with their observations until they felt that they had sufficient to produce significant results.

The second group of studies is concerned predominantly with congenital deformity. Kalick[36] studied the effects of treatment on one hundred patients with port-wine stains, but did not place them in a social context. The remaining four studies in the group were carried out at the Hospital for Sick Children in Toronto.

Lefebvre and Barclay[37] conducted a major study of the social effects of plastic surgery in 1982, with a sample of 250 patients, aged from six weeks to 39 years. Of these, 178 had congenital deformities, and 72 had acquired disfigurement; however, of these 72, 48 were concerned with prognathism or retrognathism, which are more properly classified as congenital in origin. Only 12 had tumours, and the remaining 12 had disfigurements due to accidents, inflammation, infection and burns.

Arndt et al. (the same research associates) carried out two studies published in 1986. In the first[38] they studied 22 patients, 13 girls and nine boys, aged eight to 17. Fourteen of them had severe congenital deformities, and eight had lesser problems such as malocclusion. In the same year[39], they published the results of a study of 24 children with Down's syndrome, 12 male and 12 female, aged three to seventeen. The average age was just under eight. Nineteen of the children were of school age. They were all the children of married couples, with only one child with Down's syndrome from each family. They were all Caucasian, with 41.7% resident in Toronto itself, and the remainder living in Ontario, within three hours' drive of the city. The mothers were aged 16 to 40, and the fathers were aged 21 to 44.

The remaining seven empirical studies are more directly related to the present study, being concerned with patients with cancer. Table 3.5 provides a summary of the social information provided in these seven studies. It also offers a view on its extent. Where social information is described as poor, this is because the data offered in the summary is all that there is. Where it is said to be moderate, there is a little more, and where it is described as good this is because there is at least as much information again provided in the study.

### Table 3.5
### Empirical Studies of Head and Neck Cancer

| Date | Author | Sample Numbers | Age | Gender | Social Class | Social Inf |
|------|--------|----------------|-----|--------|--------------|------------|
| 1972 | Rozen | 139 | Most 45-65 | 89 m 50 f | Most poor education | Good |
| 1973 | West | 152 | Not given | Not given | Not given | Poor |
| 1980 | Selda and Lowental | 39 | Banded 10-70 | 23 m 16 f | Race not class | Moderate |

'continued'

| 1981 | Fiegenbaum | 17 | Av. 56.2 S.D. 12.5 | Not given | Low social class, poor education | Moderate |
|------|-----------|-----|----------------------|-----------|---------------------------------|----------|
| 1982 | David and Barritt | 151 | Av. 60 | 112 m 39 f | Middle to lower | Good |
| 1984 | Morton | 48 | Over 60 | All male | Not considered | Poor |
| 1984 | Roefs | 14 | 25-73, seven over 60 | Not given | Not considered | Poor |
| 1989 | Ildstad | 542 | 19-92 | Not given | Not considered | Poor |

Rozen et al.[40] give a very clear and helpful profile of the 139 patients in their study. They described how many were indigenous to California (27%), how many had lived in the state for more than 10 years before treatment, and how many had been married for a substantial period before becoming ill. Seventy-nine percent lived with a spouse or relative. Sixty-six percent of the group were of European ethnic origin. Much additional material is provided, but it is related to the effects of surgery, and will be dealt with at that point. In conclusion, they summarise the social profile of their patients:

> ... we can describe our maxillo-facial cancer patient in the following way: he is a Caucasian man and probably 50 to 60 years of age; he is married and has had at least a high school education; he held a responsible job prior to his illness and has been able to pay most of his medical bills himself. The change from independent to dependent status accompanying his illness is evident ... Following his illness, he exhausted his emotional and financial resources, and he often receives help from State agencies and university clinics, where he pays reduced fees.[41]

Sela and Lowental[42] considered four independent variables: gender, racial origin, type of disfigurement, and age. The age distribution of the group, and of those with cancer, is given in Table 3.6.

91

### Table 3.6
### Sela and Lowental - Age Distribution    N = 39

|       | Total group | Cancer patients |
|-------|-------------|-----------------|
| 10-19 | 6           | 2               |
| 20-39 | 15          | 6               |
| 40-59 | 14          | 5               |
| 60-70 | 4           | 3               |
|       | 39          | 16              |

The authors were interested in relating the variable of racial origin to outcome. For this they distinguished only Ashkenasi Jews and non-Ashkenasi Jews, that is Jews whose parents came to Israel from Europe or North America, and Jews whose parents came from Africa or Asia. As it happened, the impact on successful prosthetic outcome was negligible. Half of the patients fell in each category.

Fiegenbaum[43], in describing a programme of rehabilitation for patients who had been treated for head and neck cancer, records little more than is described above in Table 2, but his manner of referring to the data indicates that he is fully aware of the impact of social factors on recovery and rehabilitation:

> The high average age of the clients and their low socio-economic status (blue-collar workers, low-level employees, housewives, and retirees from these professions) and low level of education (8 years as the rule) suggested action-oriented therapy elements and the use of a simple and easy to understand language.[44]

In David and Barritt's[45] description of 151 head and neck cancer patients, 83 were alive at the time of reporting, and 68 had died. The paper presents factual material about the social characteristics of the group, interwoven with comments on reactions to the illness and treatment , and commentary on the practice of the clinical team and its responses to the phenomena described. The fact that these three elements -data, general impressions, and descriptions of clinical practice - are interwoven makes it difficult to follow themes through - it would have been preferable if they had been kept discrete.

The average age of the patients was 60, and they ranged from 20 to 88. Eighty-one were city dwellers, and 70 were from small country towns. Socio-economic status in terms of "income group" - upper, middle and lower - is described in Table 3.7.

**Table 3.7**
**David and Barritt - Economic Status of Sample    N = 151**

|  | Male | Female | Total |
|---|---|---|---|
| Upper income group | 10 | 2 | 12 |
| Middle income group | 43 | 16 | 59 |
| Lower income group | 59 | 18 | 77 |

As in the present study, the largest number is from the lower social group(s), although the material is not directly comparable; the Australian study uses level of income to give a rating of social status, whereas in the British study it is derived from occupation or previous occupation.

Intake of alcohol is described in the Australian study; 57 males and eight females reported high intake of alcohol before becoming ill. Eighteen males and ten females drank little or no alcohol.

The authors draw attention to the fact that although extensive drinking outside the home may have disrupted family life, it was well established before illness. The heavy drinkers were a particularly difficult group for those concerned with rehabilitation - for example, they had little motivation to pursue speech therapy. They also reported sexual and relationship difficulties:

> Of the 93 patients with oral cancer, 27 male and three female patients had sexual problems arising out of alcoholism, which preceded the onset of the oral cancer.   These problems were well-established at the time of the initial diagnosis of cancer. These were the people who  admitted that they had marital problems. [46]

Roefs et al.'s paper[47] is included in this section because by implication their work is concerned with head and neck cancer, although they at no time say that it is so.  They refer to other works which discuss head and neck cancer, they refer to "the disease", they refer to one patient who was told about metastases in an unacceptable manner, but they do not describe their sample explicitly. Their attention to social factors is low, although they do say that "in further research, self-esteem and self-concept as well as the social

93

environment should be considered."[48]

No additional social material is available in the studies described by West, Morton et al., and Ildstad et al. This is particularly disappointing in the case of Ildstad, whose highly significant findings on survival and its association with a number of factors could usefully have been taken further.

The remaining thirteen papers reviewed in this chapter have no direct empirical base. They are based on the practice experience of their authors, within a range of settings. Five have a special significance, however, since they refer largely to the management of head and neck cancer patients - Light, Frank, Riley, Addison, and Roefs et al.

## The impact of surgery

Much of the literature focuses, quite naturally, on the results of surgery. Within this must also be taken the discussion of the consequences of prosthetic work. Increasingly over recent years, prosthetics has been superseded by more complex and skilled reconstructive surgery; more procedures have been found to be possible, more grafts of skin, tissue and bone have been carried out, and perhaps the greatest advances of all have taken place through the development of microvascular surgery; this has enabled grafts to be carried out in a single procedure, instead of the pedicle grafts previously used. For the purposes of this section, however, prosthetic reconstruction and reconstruction through live tissue are taken together.

## Positive outcomes

Arndt et al.[49] considered the impact of corrective facial surgery on a group of 22 severely or mildly disfigured children and adolescents. They found that the patients considered themselves more attractive following surgery, and that they possessed more social confidence, performing better at school, and meeting strangers in a more relaxed manner.

The appearance ratings were carried out pre-operatively, six months after surgery, and two years after surgery. It was the initial impact after surgery that produced the most significant results; for both mildly and severely affected patients the ratings had degenerated slightly by the time the two-year point was reached (the independent raters only carried out one post-operative judgement, at one year).

The study, with all its self-confessed methodological short-comings, contained important results for plastic surgeons. It emphasised the value of corrective work for young people, at a time in their lives when physical "differentness" is noted and rated negatively, by themselves and their peers.

The two main elements coming out of this study recur frequently - liking one's revised appearance, and enhanced social functioning. Kalick[50] discusses the impact of surgery upon personality, and the impact of personality on satisfaction with facial surgery. He refers to several experiments from the field of social psychology, which suggest that appearance (or believed appearance) may influence behaviour markedly. Not only will believed disfigurement induce self-consciousness, but it will affect the way in which interaction occurs. So, the two issues dealt with by Kalick are broadly those examined by Arndt et al, physical enhancement, and improved interaction. In addition, Kalick places emphasis on the personality itself, as well as on its manifestation in social interaction. Kalick's own research conflicts with many studies on patient satisfaction with patient surgery; he found that patient satisfaction correlated highly with surgical success in the treatment of part wine stains, and only very slightly with patient personality traits:

> Thus, in contrast with the common clinical folklore about patients who are unaccountably ecstatic over mediocre results or irate over good results, these systematic aggregate findings show that on the whole, with this patient sample, the patients' satisfaction is accounted for in surprising detail by what the surgeon and staff do - how considerately they treat the patient and what physical results they produce - and surprisingly little by capricious personal factors within the patient.[51]

Kalick is unreasonable to dismiss previous findings as "folklore", but his findings underline a most important factor in the determining of satisfaction, namely the nature of the original condition. The port wine stain is a definite, unequivocal congenital condition. As Kalick points out, support is usually forthcoming from family and friends to minimise maladjustment. This is in contrast to the complexity of circumstances surrounding the development of facial cancer, its treatment, and the rehabilitation of the patient, for whom appearance is only one of many concerns. In addition, while not wishing to belittle the consequences of the port wine stain to the sufferer, treatment for its removal is not necessarily so invasive as the excision of malignant facial tissue (in Kalick's study the treatment was by laser), which may result in the removal of substantial parts of the face, and which frequently require extensive reconstructive surgery.

Self-esteem and self-image are expressions used frequently by authors of works about appearance, to denote liking and valuing themselves in a range of ways, but with special regard to their body and general appearance. Lefebvre (a consultant child psychiatrist) and Barclay (a social worker) studied[52] the self-image of 250 children and adults. Patients were interviewed, and in the case of children their parents were also interviewed. Self-rating was not carried out in the case of infants, but children old enough to be interviewed yet too young to use the self-rating scale were asked to draw themselves. The majority of cases (178) were of congenital abnormality. The rest were a variety of tumours, and accidents, including burns. The average age of those presenting with congenital disorders was lower than that of the other group.

Comparisons within the total group are difficult; the disfigurements were caused in different ways; only 175 patients were able to rate themselves on the Hays self-rating scale for appearance; finally, only 125 of the patients were seen a year later. Within these constraints, nonetheless, some important results must be noted.

After surgery, in 96 out of the 125 cases seen one year later, an enhanced self-image appeared to result, together with a greater comfort when meeting others. In addition, in a further 39 of these cases an objective improvement in quality of life was reported, such as improved work performance. Some experienced no change, and some experienced increased friction in their relationships. Two patients were angry with the physical and social results of surgery.

Lefebvre and Barclay were considering three outcomes of surgery - self-image (broadly consistent with the issue of satisfaction with appearance), self-esteem (a feature of personality), and quality of life (issues of social interaction). Ratings of appearance and self-image improved after surgery, as did self-esteem. At the time of writing, There was also strong evidence that social interaction and social behaviour had improved.

Generalisations from Lefebvre and Barclay's results are difficult, because of the mixed sample which they studied -in sharp contrast to, for example, Kalick's sample of patients with port-wine stains. Another clearly-defined sample was that of Arndt et al. (2)[53], who considered the results of surgery on 24 children with Down's syndrome. In that study, outcome was evaluated almost entirely in terms of ratings of appearance - by parents and by outside evaluators. Ratings by parents are summarised in Table 3.8.

**Table 3.8**
**Arndt et al. (2) - Parent Ratings of Surgery**

|              | %     |
|--------------|-------|
| Improved     | 85.4  |
| No change    | 8.3   |
| Deteriorated | 6.3   |
|              | 100.0 |

Ratings by independent evaluators were more cautious, and far less favourable, as shown in Table 3.9.

**Table 3.9**
**Arndt et al. (2) - Independent Ratings of Surgery**

|              | %     |
|--------------|-------|
| Improved     | 18.3  |
| No change    | 27.9  |
| Deteriorated | 53.8  |
|              | 100.0 |

These findings suggest that the felt improvement is more important than actual objective measurement, especially as family functioning was also reported to be healthy after surgery:

> The fact that half of them chose to continue to procreate after the birth of their Down syndrome child shows an optimistic attitude. In family functioning, the parents' self-reports were remarkably similar to the norms. The report of slightly more cohesion on the FACES Scale after surgery may reflect a unifying effect on the family by the surgery.[54]

## Negative outcomes and costs

Riley, in his paper on the classification of maxillo-facial prostheses, makes full acknowledgement of the psychological impact on the patient of the loss of tissue through cancer:

> The loss of an ear, nose, eye, or parts of the palate presents a psychologic, functional, and aesthetic burden that is difficult for the average individual to accept. It is also an economic and sociologic crisis if the deformity precludes the patient's gainful employment.[55]

A substantial part of the literature on head and neck cancer is concerned with its negative consequences - with the illness itself, with the consequences of mutilation caused by surgery, and with practical resultant difficulties. Rozen et al.'s follow up study[56] describes these three features. The questionnaires completed for this study were administered in an interview shortly after the rehabilitation process had begun. In this way, and in terms of the subject matter covered in the interviews, there are strong similarities to the present study.

In Rozen et al.'s study, one of the most serious problems encountered by clinic staff was depression, originating from fears surrounding the disease itself, and from the deteriorated self-image which it induced, but also compounded by communication problems. A variety of forms of therapy were used in order to enhance the patients' emotional, social and vocational functioning.

Morton et al.[57] stressed the need to consider the emotional and social costs of treatment, in addition to accustomed measures of success; traditionally, cancer treatment is evaluated by such measures as survival time and remission, and no one would discount their primacy; however, the authors note the trend amongst oncologists of considering the patient's quality of life as a result of intervention. Their study of 48 elderly men treated in Liverpool for cancer involving the cheek and/or throat examined eight aspects of current well-being, covering functional, emotional and cosmetic aspects of living.

Generally, those treated by radiotherapy had adjusted to life better than those who had undergone surgery. The latter performed better in functional terms, but they were less satisfied with their bodies. In the measures of emotional well-being, there was no difference between the two groups, and the overall level of depression was high, at 39%. The results might suggest that patients view surgery as more invasive than radiotherapy, and therefore as more destructive to the self.

The sample was one with extremely well-defined boundaries - the subjects were all male, over 60 years old, retired, who had buccopharyngeal cancer, with no manifestation over the previous six months. Although this undoubtedly assisted the evaluation of the results, cross-study comparisons might be difficult, since few studies will have restricted the social characteristics of their group to the same extent. In addition, "quality of life" covers a range of factors, and it is unlikely that many studies will apply the same measures.

The authors suggest that as different forms of treatment produce different results, the determinants of quality of life are likely to be multiple rather than unidimensional. However, the findings would indicate that the illness itself causes mood difficulties, but the treatment is disabling, affecting personal and social performance subsequently.

This is borne out by Sela and Lowental[58], of the Hadassah University Hospital, Jerusalem, who carried out a study of the outcome of facial prosthetic treatment. They examined the psychological well-being of patients who were fitted with a facial prosthesis - looking at areas of psychological functioning as a measure of successful outcome rather than the patients' statements of satisfaction with or acceptance of the device.

The authors had expected that age and ethnic origin would influence psychological functioning. In fact they did not do so. They found that the only variation for age was in early adolescence. As far as ethnic difference is concerned, Sela and Lowental's sample was an all-Jewish group, and the only ethnic distinction was between Ashkenasi Jews - whose parents had come from Europe and America - and non-Ashkenasi Jews - whose parents had come from Asia and Africa. Broader ethnic differences might have produced different results.

Thirty-three of the 39 subjects had improved their ratings in aspects such as self-image and feelings of health. Those who had responded best were patients who had become disfigured as a result of trauma. The second most improved group was that of congenitally deformed patients, and those least improved were those whose disfigurement had arisen from malignancy. As explanation of these differences, the authors say:

> ... many of the cancer patients have an inner feeling of being doomed, despite all modern successful therapy and the remission achieved; their restored external appearance cannot rectify their feelings. People who have an accidental trauma, on the other hand, even if wounded or maimed, do not develop a

similar conviction ... most of them retain their normal drives for health and for rehabilitation, and a prosthetic restoration of their appearance facilitates their progress.[59]

In his address to the New York State Medical Society in 1979, Professor Stephen Nordlicht[60] considered the role of the psychiatrist in the management of facial cancer, describing some of the psychiatric factors which may be involved. He emphasised the complexity of feelings which may result from facial disfigurement, because of the importance of the face as the location of the sensory organs, as well as being an indicator of finer feelings. Nordlicht therefore focuses on the second of the two negative features, appearance resulting from mutilating surgery.

Depression may result from the disfigurement, and may be aggravated by difficulties which existed prior to the facial loss. The loss may leave a permanently vulnerable personality, and in Nordlicht's view psychiatric oversight is indicated in all cases. He describes the process of acceptance of change, from superficial acceptance, to denial, and finally acceptance and adjustment. There is always the possibility of serious reaction, and care must be taken to counsel the patient and his family. Loneliness must be avoided, as this places the patient at emotional risk, sometimes predisposing him to suicide. On discharge, help must be given with rehabilitation, as the patient's problems are only beginning when he steps outside the hospital.

Nordlicht's views represent advice rather than evidence. Generally, he is right to be cautious about the patient's ability to adjust, but perhaps because of his professional position he places more emphasis than many on the need for psychiatric oversight. It could well be argued that there is a range of reactions to disfiguring surgery which come within the range of normal, and others which are abnormal. It is this latter group which psychiatrists might most usefully assist, and they could reasonably rely on referrals from other professionals to do so - surgeons, nurses, physiotherapists, social workers and occupational therapists.

By far the most comprehensive approach to the consequences of facial surgery through cancer is taken by David and Barritt,[61] a social worker and a plastic surgeon. They consider in particular detail the practical difficulties faced by patients during rehabilitation.

First of all, in relation to cancer itself, David and Barritt looked at alcohol abuse particularly as a feature of becoming ill, since excessive alcohol consumption is strongly associated with head and neck cancer.

In their Australian study, 57 males and eight females reported high intake of alcohol before becoming ill. Eighteen males and ten females drank little or no alcohol. Following surgery, ten of the 57 males, and two of the eight females, ceased drinking. No one increased their consumption.

All patients in their study underwent substantial emotional upheaval. Many reacted very emotionally to the diagnosis, and post-operative depression occurred in all patients, but was particularly severe for the ten patients for whom an endogenous element already existed. Fear of death was also widely reported, and the sensation of becoming aware of the closeness of death.

Several people (an unspecified number) found that change in their facial appearance was a problem. They were appalled at the mutilation, they were terrified by the need to acquire a new body image, and afraid of how they were going to adapt their life to suit their changed appearance following survival.

David and Barritt described a range of practical difficulties encountered by the recovering head and neck cancer patient, which are summarised as follows:

- There was a two-fold financial problem - lower income, and shorter earning life;
- The social value of the face and mouth was highlighted by their distortion - they are required for adequate performance in communication and social functioning such as eating together;
- The illness and treatment imposed stresses and difficulties on family life;
- Dependency on the treatment centre was a marked phenomenon. In South Australia, many patients live a long way from the treatment centre, and this provokes a fear of isolation from vital sources of help;
- Controlling pain, and overcoming practical difficulties, including speaking, swallowing, and reducing offensive odours. All of these have emotional and social aspects to them, in addition to them being a practical issue.

David and Barritt could have provided more quantifiable material on reactions to illness, surgery and disfigurement; it is unclear whether the characteristics described are majority or minority observations. Nonetheless, valuable insights are provided, both into the disorder, and into professional responses to it.

## Indicators for successful surgery

Lefebvre and Munro[62] considered from a psychiatric perspective the impact of surgery on children who have severe facial deformities, and on their families. Lefebvre and Munro were particularly interested to know whether there was a preferred time in a child's life to operate, what the overall impact of surgery was on the child, and what psychological factors might suggest that the child should not undergo surgery.

Although it had been expected that results would suggest that surgery should be performed as early as technically possible, this was not the case. However, it is difficult to know what exactly the authors mean when they say that "....the two critical considerations should be the readiness of the parents and the child's expectations."

Although one of the aims of the study was to learn what the physical, psychological and social impact was of surgery, this occupies a very small part. All that is said is that the results of surgery were physically good, and that there was enhanced social performance. More emphasis is placed on a description of the impact of the original deformity on the lives of the children.

The principal positive indicators for surgery are that parents and child should both understand what is involved and want it very much, but dissatisfaction is high when the child is subjected to parental pressure to have surgery. Other contraindications, such as previous psychological malfunctioning, were not seen as impediments to successful outcome.

It might be argued that the results of Lefebvre and Munro's study are not readily transferable to the context of adult head and neck cancer. Perhaps of more relevance are the findings of Roefs et al., who were dealing with prosthetic rehabilitation, rather than purely with reconstruction. Roefs et al.[63], at the University of Groningen in the Netherlands, found in a small sample of patients (14) who regularly visited their department for management of a prosthesis that the strongest determinant of acceptance of the prosthesis by the patient (which was considered as the most important measure of its effectiveness) was not its "objectively" assessed quality. Their prostheses were rated by the authors for their "form, colour, translucency, retention and concealment". Little association was found between these "objective" ratings and the patients' "subjective" acceptance of the prostheses. Although the skills of the maxillo-facial technician are important in the rehabilitation of the patient who requires a facial prosthesis, the aesthetic quality of a prosthesis is not the strongest determinant of its effectiveness.

In a series of interviews with the patients, variables were considered which might influence acceptance of the prosthesis - particularly the patient's social environment, the doctor-patient relationship, and the nature of the defect. Factors which had been thought to influence acceptance were not found to be reliable. The authors suggest that there was some evidence from the interviews that "self-concept" was more influential.

The authors are cautious about their findings, partly because of the small numbers, and partly because the interviews were conducted in the clinic, by clinic staff. Their findings in relation to influential factors are inconclusive, but those concerned with evaluation of the prosthesis are of importance. They would suggest that it is only valuable to a certain point to concentrate on improving the actual prosthesis. Thereafter, the bulk of effort needs to be towards encouraging the individual's confidence.

If indeed the findings of Roefs et al. may be applied to plastic surgery as well as to artificial replacement, the emphasis during the rehabilitation phase needs to be placed at least as much on the confidence of the individual as on the actual technical levels of achievement. This will be addressed again in a later chapter.


**Facing the future**

For those who have undergone head and neck surgery, questions about the future are clearly divided into two groups: first, questions about survival, and second, questions about rehabilitation - what helps people survive, and what helps them to lead a fuller life.

As Sela and Lowental assert, feelings of being doomed outweigh all other considerations for head and neck cancer patients. The authors assert that, unlike other patients who present for head and neck surgery, cancer patients have lost their will to achieve health. The present study is not intended as an epidemiological survey, but when the question of head and neck cancer is being discussed, the issue of survival cannot be ignored. While the sample is small, nonetheless what conclusions may be drawn will be highlighted.

In the study by David and Barritt of a group of head and neck cancer patients in Australia, survival is referred to obliquely, by virtue of their description of the proportion of the sample alive at the time of writing -55%. However, it is difficult to draw any conclusions from the reference, as a basic description of their methodology is lacking.

A more systematic approach was taken by Ildstad et al.,[64] who considered the possible characteristics which influence the survival of patients with head and neck cancer, by means of a regression analysis of 542 patients. The factor which most influenced survival was the tumour stage at the point of presentation. Advanced age and location of the tumour in the tonsillar area were also associated with poor survival. Type of therapy and gender were not significant. Factors concerned with survival will be addressed when presenting the findings from the present study.

Having survived, the patient must then aim to recover normal conditions of living - recovery from illness, and adaptation to a revised appearance. West[65] studied 152 patients recovering from head and neck surgery, in order to see what causes people to adapt well to acquired disfigurement. He found that most had adapted well, and names four factors which influenced this. The first was age; the patients were quite old, and therefore well-established within their community. Secondly, they had all survived cancer, and relief which this caused was uppermost in their minds. Third, they appeared to have had a good hospital experience, and finally, the group was otherwise representative of the wider, "normal" population; the assumption is that apart from their illness they had no more problems than anyone else. The sample was relatively large (152) and the results are credible.

West found that patients who had a good body image adapted well to their revised appearance. Other positive indicators were an attitude of working to overcome the disease and return to the community, high family expectations and support, and a high level of social contact. Given the emphasis on staying in touch with people, it is consistent that those with speech difficulties did not adjust well. (This is reinforced by Van Doorne, who stated that prostheses which facilitate eating and speaking are accepted more readily than those which are extra-oral, and only cosmetic.)

There are clear messages here for those assisting the recovery of head and neck cancer patients, and also strong links with the present study, in which most of the survivors have resumed their previous settled way of life. The principal message is that to settle back into normal life after surgery, one needs to have had a settled life in the first place. If that condition is fulfilled, such patients are likely to have no greater social problems generally than any other group of people.

## What can be done?

Much advice is given in these papers to professionals on how to help the social and psychological functioning of patients after surgery. For example, Friedenbergs[66], as a result of his study of the psychological impact of skin cancers at the New York Institute of Rehabilitative Medicine, produced a very down-to-earth set of precepts for clinical practitioners:

- Dermatologists should not assume that patients concerned with minor facial lesions are narcissistic;
- Patients may believe (rightly on occasions) that skin cancers are life-threatening, and the doctor should elicit what the patient understands of their condition;
- Patients should be advised of the dangers of comparing their condition to that of others;
- Indications for referral to a mental health professional would include the following:
- If the patient asks for it or is unduly upset;
- Obvious psychiatric symptoms;
- Impairment of everyday functioning;
- Interference with medical treatment;
- Greater pain than one would normally associate with the condition;
- Certain life-threatening lesions of the face or neck.

From the perspective of the psychiatrist, although addressing maxillo-facial technicians, Frank[67], himself a psychiatrist, offers advice on how to empathise with the withdrawn patient, enabling him or her to express painful feelings. The technician is in a good position to do so, "... since he is seen as being a person who provides practical help in the problems of re-adjustment." The practice experience on which Frank draws is no doubt substantial, but the paper says nothing new, and also appears to talk down to the maxillo-facial technician; the latter is counselled that he or she is not a psychological expert, although still of use to the patient:

> ... if he reinforces the empathy and understanding of an intelligent layman with experience and a little knowledge, he will be highly effective ...[68]

Addison, a social worker, speaking at the same conference for maxillo-facial technicians, offered a theoretical framework for understanding loss, and derived several precepts which could be of use in working with those who have lost facial tissue. Addison, who at the time of writing was a social worker at the Queen Mary Hospital, Roehampton, suggests that acceptance of the disfigurement and tolerance of the prosthesis is a grieving process, which will require working through the same stages of recovery as for any other serious loss. The disfigured person must carry out this recovery without the benefit of the public rites of passage which accompany bereavement by death. The comparison is more than allegorical, and it therefore follows that:

- Previously low self-image will be even lower after disfigurement;
- A period of mourning is needed, before any impression is formed of psychological surgical results of surgery;
- Space must be allowed for the patient to give vent to anger;
- And finally, the pain which staff may experience must be acknowledged.

More specific approaches are offered by Fiegenbaum, and by Roback et al, on how to help the patient who needs encouragement, training or other help to become confident in dealing with others. Fiegenbaum[69], of the Philipps University of Marburg, West Germany, studied the value of behaviour therapy to assist in the enhancement of the daily living skills of patients who undergo facial surgery, using patients from the Otolaryngology Clinic at the University of Cologne.

A total of 17 patients, all of whom had had face or neck surgery from cancer during the previous four years, participated in a social training programme whose aim was to encourage patients to develop active strategies to solve problems generated by their disfigurement. The study then evaluated the training, using as measures of success the following factors:

1. Self-confidence;
2. Anxiety in making contact with people;
3. Anxiety in particular social settings, and
4. Self-image

Fiegenbaum summarised the problems which facial cancer patients may experience:

... social anxiety, lack of self-confidence, negative self-image, behaviour deficits, depressive reactions up to suicide, drug addiction, aggression, increased sensibility or irritability, total adaptation and overcompensation.[70]

This impressive list of possible pathological reactions is derived totally from quoted sources. Recovery from both the physical condition and its psychosocial consequences is further impeded by fear of further onset of malignant growth.

Consequently it was thought worthwhile to develop specific rehabilitative techniques relevant to the age group (predominantly 55 to 60) and cross-section of social class distribution of facial cancer patients.

Before and after a period of social training, the subjects' social performance was evaluated. After this very practical and relevant series of sessions, substantial improvement had been achieved in the fields of anxiety level and self-confidence, but no actual improvement was achieved in the actual image which the individual had of himself or herself.

The study provides very practical guidance to professionals, principally to the effect that counselling should be conducted both before and after surgery, ranging from ensuring that the patient is fully aware of what is happening to him or her, through to the treatment of severe abreactions.

Roback et al.[71] at the Vanderbilt University School of Medicine described the situation of a man affected in a very mild way by neurofibromatosis. Unlike the most well-known person with that disorder - the "Elephant Man" - in this person's case the disorder was restricted to a cyst on the face, and small multiple growths on one arm. He had previously had other tumours removed surgically. His confidence in his own ability to relate to others was low, and he underwent a programme to enhance his communication skills:

> Objectively, his physical disfigurement was slight, and unlikely to account fully for his social ineffectiveness. Rather, it appeared that through his relative isolation and the ways he viewed himself in relation to others, he had never learned how to communicate effectively.[72]

Much of the communication skills programme focused on the man's aspirations to ask out a woman with whom he worked, and by the end of the therapy he had both accepted that this was not going to happen, and established a sound and valued friendship with her.

From this study the authors draw the important general point that people with a congenital deformity gain much of their self-concept in relation to the disfigurement from their parents, whereas those who are disfigured later in life, when they have established their own view of what they look like, and who they are, make their own judgement about the effect of their disfigurement. Consequently, the authors' advice to therapists working with those with a congenital disfigurement is that where possible they work with the whole family unit.

The case illustration is clearly presented, and the conclusions drawn are reasonable and well argued; the article is a useful contribution to professional practice.

Rehabilitation of cancer patients with the assistance of prosthetics is discussed by Cordell Riley, of the University of California School of Dentistry.[73] This is an early work, describing greater reliance on prosthetics than would be acceptable at the present time, when techniques of reconstructive surgery are better developed.

The preferred means of correction of facial disfigurement, however caused, is plastic surgery, but in some situations this would prove ill-advised, or impossible. Riley describes the circumstances in which a facial prosthesis would be indicated. His classification is still valid, although those within each category might be less, as plastic surgery has become viable for more people:

> (1) in the very old patients, (2) in those without sufficient time or funds for multiple plastic procedures, (3) in those with exceptionally large defects, (4) in those in whom the local tissue has a diminished blood supply due to irradiation, and (5) in those whose post-operative defects are being observed for possible tumour recurrence. In these situations, a removable prosthesis is the treatment of choice.[74]

The contribution of prosthetics to rehabilitation is seen as substantial, but it must be seen within the context of the patient's overall well-being:

> The patient who must be subjected to radical surgery is in need of complete understanding and sympathy. Every means to assist the patient to rapid recovery and rehabilitation should be explored. This consideration for the patient is as important as the operation itself.[75].

The principal focus for Riley is technical, and the article is a most useful summary of types of prosthesis, temporary and more permanent, including those used in the course of reconstructive surgery; many of the techniques described are still in use. In addition, however, this article also offers a useful illustration of a clinician taking a broader view of patient well-being than the purely technical one.

It is therefore suggested that cancer patients need special attention, and the nature of the help referred to, but not described in detail:

> Cancer patients, especially those who appear introverted, may require a psychiatric consultation, but often the dentist in charge will succeed through his own humanistic orientation.[76]

This is presuming much. Without going into more detailed investigation, it cannot be said that the needs of introverted cancer patients can best be met by a psychiatrist. Nor can it always be assumed that the surgeon's own "humanistic orientation" - if indeed he has one - will be of value to the remainder; how will it help? The research finding that cancer patients are vulnerable, or at least do not function so well, is valuable, but the same rigour which has been applied to describing the problem should be given to its solution.

Sela and Lowental's contribution to the discussion on rehabilitation is also concerned with prosthetics, but it is less than helpful. It is based on a pathological view of the patient and his or her ability to recover from serious illness and surgery. The authors state that psychiatric assessment is required in most cases of people with head and neck cancer. The case is not argued, and ignores the inherent strength of the individual to recover from major physical and emotional upheaval.

Several of the authors emphasise the need for inter-disciplinary collaboration. Light[77] reviewed some of the available psychosocial material, and asserted that some of the negative social and psychological features associated with facial cancer surgery could be offset by the close cooperation of a multi-disciplinary team. He referred to the complexity of problems of those requiring facial surgery, and set the skills of the surgeon within their social context:

> We have succeeded in increasing the survival rate of individuals with cancer of the head and neck by applying modern techniques of radical orificial surgery. Although the life span of these patients has been lengthened, problems remain. They may have to contend with severe cosmetic

disfigurements and functional defects in speech, mastication, swallowing and salivary control. Such physical handicaps cannot be masked or hidden. Moreover, they remain secondary to social and psychological disabilities which may prove an even greater barrier to successful rehabilitation.[78]

A plea for the professions to collaborate closely, and work as a team, is made by Ian Munro[79], in an article written whilst he was practising at the Hospital for Sick Children in Toronto. Munro argued that a team approach to facial surgery was the only effective one, and furthermore such teams should be organised on a regional basis, to enable sufficient experience to be developed within the team. He recommended that the team should include a broad range of clinical and non-clinical professionals, listing fourteen different professionals in all, ranging from the plastic surgeon to the medical illustrator. The team would include a substantial psycho-social component, whose role would be two-fold: its members should assess the patient and family before surgery, in order to gauge how well the trauma was likely to be tolerated. They would also help the patient post-operatively to adjust to the new role into which the revised facial image would cast him or her, and help him or her overcome other hurdles of re-integration as they occurred.

David and Barritt give a clear picture of the work of the multi-disciplinary team. Heavy emphasis is placed on the need for inter-disciplinary co-operation at all stages, with the surgeon acting as team leader and co-ordinator of community medical services, and the hospital social worker acting as co-ordinator both within the hospital team and amongst professionals in the community.

A psycho-social assessment is conducted pre-operatively and three months after surgery, and thereafter as required. The pre-operative interview is carried out by the surgeon and social worker. In addition the intensive care staff and post-operative ward staff meet the patient before theatre. Before discharge the team prepares the patient and his or her family to be aware of the particular problems likely to be encountered, and how to overcome them.

Following discharge, a full multi-disciplinary assessment is carried out at three months. The patient (with family) is also seen at regular out-patient appointments, where any additional difficulties may be reported.

The surgical team is constantly under pressure to improve its techniques, partly because of its own wish to raise standards, and partly because of the wishes of patients to improve their appearance.

## Conclusions

1. The contributions to the literature on facial disfigurement and facial surgery are predominantly from the clinical and therapeutic professions. The material quite understandably takes on some of the flavour of the discipline of the author; this is particularly so in the case of psychiatrists, who by the very nature of their specialism focus on psychopathology.

2. The work of Bull and his associates illustrates and confirms that facially disfigured people are shunned by others and disadvantaged socially. The importance of the face in social relations is emphasised by others, and consequently any facial impairment poses a threat to emotional and social equilibrium.

3. The characteristics of those who are disfigured through surgery in order to alleviate facial cancer have been described whenever this has been a feature in a study; the patients tend to be of lower social classes, more male than female, and in late middle age, with a tendency to smoke and to drink heavily. This has been common to studies in the United States, the U.K. and Australia.

4. Surgery to correct congenital deformity tends to be successful: assuming that the actual surgery is of sufficient quality, the correction caused people to feel more attractive, and to perform more confidently in social situations. On the other hand, surgery which has had to be performed because of head and neck cancer is accompanied by negative features - depression, dissatisfaction with the body, reduction in quality of life, and family tensions. This may be associated in part with the illness itself, but those treated for head and neck cancer less invasively, by radiotherapy, were not so badly affected. Generally, those whose ego strengths were strong and intact prior to illness functioned better afterwards, along with older people with a settled way of life, and people with good family support networks.

5. Cancer of the head and neck is very life-threatening. Long term survival rates are poor, and are influenced by a number of factors: the most at risk are older people, those who do not seek help early enough, and those whose tumour is in the

tonsillar area.

6.	There is much that professionals can do to alleviate the social consequences of facial surgery. The first is to gain an understanding of the consequences of the disfigurement to the person. This will assist in developing an empathetic approach to whatever course of treatment or therapy is being offered. A range of therapies is described; they include psychiatric management of depression, and behaviour therapy (both group and individual) to increase confidence and social skills. Several authors stress the need for professions to work together, to identify and reduce risk to the recovering patient. The sum of their viewpoints is felt to be substantially more valuable than when they work separately and independently.

**Notes**

1.	Rozen, R.D., Ordway, D.E., Curtis, T.A., and Cantor, R., 1972, 'Psychosocial aspects of maxillo-facial rehabilitation. Part 1. The effect of primary cancer treatment,' *The Journal of Prosthetic Dentistry,* October, 28, 4, pp. 423-428.
2.	David, D.J. and Barritt, J.A., 1982, 'Psychosocial implications of surgery for head and neck cancer', *Clinics in Plastic Surgery*, 9,3, July.
3.	Ildstad, S., Tollerud, D.J., Bigelow, M.E., and Remensnyder, J.P., 1989, 'A multivariate analysis of determinants of survival for patients with squamous cell carcinoma of the head and neck,' *Ann. Surg.*, February, 209, 2, pp. 237-241.
4.	Roback, H.B., Kirshner, and Roback, E., 1981-2, 'Physical self-concept changes in a mildly facially disfigured neurofibromatosis patient following communication skill training', *International Journal of Psychiatry in Medicine*, 11, 2, pp. 137-143.
5.	Kalick, S.M., 1982, 'Clinician, Social Scientist and Body Image', *Clinics in Plastic Surgery* 9, 3, pp. 379-385, July.
6.	Constable, J.D. and Bernstein, N.R., 1979, 'Public and professional reactions to the facially disfigured which interfere with rehabilitation,' *Scandinavian Journal of Plastic and Reconstructive Surgery*, 13, 1, pp. 181-183.
7.	Van Doorne, J., 1981, 'Psychosocial aspects of cancer patients with facial disfigurement,' *International Facial Prosthetic Workshop*, pp. 80-88.

8.   Peterson, L.J., and Topazian, R.G., 1974, 'The preoperative interview and psychological evaluation of the orthognathic surgery patient', *Journal of Oral Surgery*, 32, 8, pp. 583-588.

9.   op. cit., p. 583.

10.  Addison, C., 1975, 'Social aspects of facial prosthetics', *International Prosthetic Workshop, Part I*, Institute of Maxillo-facial Technology, pp. 146-152.

11.  Frank, O.S., 1975, 'Psychosocial factors in the prosthetic rehabilitation of the facially disfigured patient', presented at the *International Facial Prosthetic Workshop*, Institute of Maxillo-facial Technology, pp. 142-145.

12.  op. cit., p. 145.

13.  ibid.

14.  Nordlicht, S., 1979, 'Facial disfigurement and psychiatric sequelae', *New York State Journal of Medicine*, 79, 9, pp. 1382-1384.

15.  Bull, R., and Stevens, J., 1981, 'The effects of facial disfigurement on helping behaviour', *The Italian Journal of Psychology*, Vol. viii, No. 1, April.

16.  Bull, R., and Stevens, J., 1981, 'The relationship between ratings of persons' facial appearance and ratings of their conversations', *Language and Speech*, Vol. 24, Part 3.

17.  Rumsey, N., Bull, R., and Gahagan, D., 1982, 'The effect of facial disfigurement on the proxemic behaviour of the general public', *Journal of Applied Social Psychology*, 12, 2, pp. 1397-150.

18.  op. cit., p. 137.

19.  op. cit., p. 148.

20.  Rumsey, N., Bull, R., and Gahagan, D., 1986, 'A developmental study of children's stereotyping of facially deformed adults', *British Journal of Psychology*, 77, pp. 269-274.

21.  Bull, R., 1982, 'Physical Appearance and Criminality', *Current Psychological Reviews*, 2, pp. 269-282.

22.  Addison, C., op. cit.

23.  Constable, J.D., and Bernstein, N.R., op. cit.

24.  op. cit., p. 181.

25.  Bailey, L.W., and Edwards, D, 1975, 'Psychological considerations in maxillo-facial prosthetics', *Journal of Prosthetic Dentistry*, 34, 5, pp. 533-538.

26.  op. cit., p. 534.

27.  ibid.

28. op. cit., p. 536.
29. Stricker, G., et al., 1979, 'Psychosocial aspects of craniofacial disfigurement', *American Journal of Orthodontics*, 76, 4, pp. 410-422.
30. op. cit., p. 412.
31. ibid.
32. op. cit., p. 416.
33. Lefebvre, A., and Barclay, S., 1982, 'Psychosocial impact of craniofacial deformities before and after reconstructive surgery', *Canadian Journal of Psychiatry*, 27, 7, pp. 579-584.
34. Riley, C., 1968, 'Maxillo-facial prosthetic rehabilitation of postoperative cancer patients', *Journal of Prosthetic Dentistry*, October, 20, 4, pp. 352-360.
35. op. cit., p. 352.
36. Kalick, op. cit.
37. Lefebvre and Barclay, op. cit.
38. Arndt, E.M., Travis, F., Lefebvre, A., Nice, A., and Munro, I.R., 1986, 'Beauty and the eye of the beholder: social consequences and personal adjustment of facial patients', *British Journal of Plastic Surgery*, 39, pp. 81-84.
39. Arndt, E.M., Lefebvre, A., Travis, F., and Munro, I.R., 1986, 'Fact and fantasy: psychosocial consequences of facial surgery in 24 Downs Syndrome children', *British Journal of Plastic Surgery*, 39, pp. 498-504.
40. Rozen et al., op. cit.
41. op. cit., p. 426.
42. Sela, M., and Lowental, U., 1980, 'Therapeutic effects of maxillo-facial prostheses', *Oral Surgery*, July, 50, 1, pp. 13-16.
43. Fiegenbaum, W., 1981, 'A social training program for clients with facial disfigurations: a contribution to the rehabilitation of cancer patients', *International Journal of Rehabilitation Research*, 4 (4), pp. 501-509.
44. op. cit., p. 504.
45. David, D.J., and Barritt, J.A., op. cit.
46. op. cit., p. 332.
47. Roefs, A.J.M., van Oort, R.P., and Schaub, R.M.H., 1984, 'Factors related to the acceptance of facial prostheses', *The Journal of Prosthetic Dentistry*, Dec. 52, 6, pp. 849-852.
48. op. cit., p. 851.
49. Arndt et al., op. cit. (1).
50. Kalick, S.M., op. cit.
51. op cit., p. 383.

52. Lefebvre,A., and Barclay, S, op. cit.
53. Arndt et al., op. cit. (2).
54. op. cit., p. 502.
55. Riley, C., op. cit., p. 352.
56. Rozen et al., op. cit.
57. Morton, R.P. et al., 1984, 'Quality of life in treated head and neck cancer patients', *Clinical Otolaryngology*, 9, 3, pp. 81-185.

58. Sela, M., and Lowental, U., op. cit.
59. op. cit., p. 15.
60. Nordlicht, S., 1979, 'Facial disfigurement and psychiatric sequelae', *New York State Journal of Medicine*, 79, 9, pp. 1382-1384.
61. David and Barritt, op. cit.
62. Lefebvre, A., and Munro, I.R., 1978, 'The role of psychiatry in a craniofacial team', *Plastic and Reconstructive Surgery*, April 61, 4, pp. 564-56.
63. Roefs, A.J.M., van Oort, R.P., and Schaub, R.M.H., 1984, 'Factors related to the acceptance of facial prostheses', *The Journal of Prosthetic Dentistry*, Dec. 52, 6, pp. 849-852.
64. Ildstad et al., op. cit.
65. West, D.W., 1973, 'Adaptation to surgically induced facial disfigurement among cancer patients, referred to in 1974, *Dissertation Abstracts International*, 34, 7, p. 4442.
66. Friedenbergs, I., 1981, 'Psychosocial management of patients with cutaneous cancers', *Journal of Dermatologic Surgery and Oncology*, 7, 10, pp. 323-330.
67. Frank, op. cit.
68. Frank, op. cit., p. 145.
69. Fiegenbaum, W., 1981, 'A social training program for clients with facial disfigurations: a contribution to the rehabilitation of cancer patients', *International Journal of Rehabilitation Research*, 4 (4), pp. 501-509.
70. op. cit., p. 503.
71. Roback, H.B., Kirshner, and Roback, E., 1981-2, 'Physical self-concept changes in a mildly facially disfigured neurofibromatosis patient following communication skill training', *International Journal of Psychiatry in Medicine*, 11, 2, pp. 137-143.
72. op. cit., p. 138.
73. Riley, C., op. cit.
74. Op. cit., p. 352.
75. ibid.

76. Op. cit., p. 359.
77. Light, J., 1976, 'Psychological aspects of disability and rehabilitation of cancer patients', *New York Journal of Dentistry*, 46, 9, November, pp. 293-297.
78. op. cit., p. 293.
79. Munro, I.R., 1975, 'Orbito-cranio-facial surgery: the team approach', *Plastic and Reconstructive Surgery*, February, 55, 2, pp. 170-176.

# 4 Voices of experience

So far the literature which has been surveyed has been written by professionals - a range of helpers, curers and research staff concerned with one or more aspect of deformity or disfigurement. There also exists a small body of literature on individuals who suffer or who have suffered disfigurement. One well-known story is that of the "Elephant Man", an individual afflicted with severe neurofibromatosis.[1]

The three principal books reviewed in this chapter are all autobiographies, describing the experiences of three very different people, and their responses to disfigurement. James Partridge described his experience of injury and burning in a car accident, and from his own experience developed a framework of advice and guidance for others. Simon Weston talked about his experience when the Sir Galahad was bombed during the Falklands War. He is also concerned to describe how he became disfigured and disabled during the attack, and how he recovered from the ensuing injury and depression. Christine Piff told how she was found to have facial cancer, how she was treated, and how she recovered. The treatment itself was mutilating, and she reacted in a most distinctive way to being disfigured by forming a UK-wide organisation of those who have been disfigured in any way.

## James Partridge

"Changing Faces - The Challenge of Facial Disfigurement"[2] was written by James Partridge, farmer, teacher of economics, writer, broadcaster and former health economics research worker. Partridge was severely burned in a road traffic accident when he was aged eighteen, twenty years before the publication of this book in 1990.[3]

"Changing Faces" is addressed to those who are disfigured for life, and for those who know someone who is disfigured; its purpose is to show that one can come to terms with disfigurement, and live a normal life. (Partridge uses the expression "changing faces" to describe this "coming to terms". Like Goffman, from whom he draws some of his material, he introduces his own specially-defined terminology.) The book is also intended to provide useful insights for professionals in health care.

According to its author, this is not an autobiographical work, but it is clear that his own experience is the starting point for much of what he says, and for his reflections on disfigurement, clinical treatment, and successful rehabilitation. For example, his chapter on facing up to the origins of disfigurement begins with a series of descriptions of and reflections on the experience of being burned.

The work is in two parts. The first, "Reconstructing Your Face", is concerned with treatment, both acute and longer-term reconstructive surgery. In practice, many of the precepts contained in this section come too late for the person who is undergoing emergency treatment for newly-sustained injuries or illness; he or she would have had no opportunity to read the advice on how first to look in the mirror, or how to assist close relatives when they first have sight of one's revised appearance. Indeed they might be physically unable to do so. However, the section would be of immense value to professionals.


## Communication

A precept which is aimed particularly at surgeons is that they should acquire communication skills:

> The surgeon should have qualifications in 'communication skills' along with his medical training, and set the tone for your facial rehabilitation by being available for lengthy conversations when necessary...[4]

How realistic this is is debatable, but Partridge is adamant that "Language training should be part of the treatment package in every burns unit...".[5] In addition to the patient's need to know what is happening to ensure their well-being, the author is also concerned that the patient should stay in control of his or her own future - "You hold the reins!".[6] Several examples are cited (from his own experience[7]) of challenges to the power and mystery of the medical profession. As part of the process of challenging, he advises that the patient must get to know clinical terminology, for example the classification of skin grafts and flaps. It must be said that this was his own experience, and it may not work for everyone. He is a highly intelligent professional person, with a background in health care (albeit inspired by his own clinical condition), and it may be beyond the ability or aspiration of the average patient. The patients in the present study are predominantly working-class people, and it may be placing unreasonable demands on them. Perhaps the onus should be on the surgeon to describe procedures in non-technical language. Partridge himself risks being accused of mystifying on occasions, such as his reference to "hypertrophic scarring".[8] Generally, in this section, the author is asking much of the patient - putting visitors at their ease, asking for clinical terms to be explained, and assisting the surgeon in pacing the treatment. He was an intelligent person, about to go up to Oxford, and allowance must be made for those who do not have his gifts or privileges.

The issue of honesty to the patient is discussed, and the conclusion is reached that the truth must be filtered on occasions in order to encourage the patient and family to maintain optimism.[9] This is a much debated issue, and it is difficult to reach a universal conclusion, but in suggesting that on occasions the hospital staff know best, and that they must err on the positive side, Partridge seems to be qualifying his exhortation to patients that they should stay in control of their own treatment. It is a useful qualifier, acknowledging the weakness and vulnerability experienced during the early stages of treatment.


**Professional help**

The contribution of other professionals is given substantial attention. It would appear that the author had a good relationship with physiotherapists, as they are given frequently as the illustration of a good listening ear (so is the ward cleaner). In this and in the second part of the book, the role of the psychologist is described, in terms of normal psychology, and their value emphasised as a means of expressing safely the powerful emotions which the patient is likely to experience. The value of social workers is often emphasised, but their role is never fully defined. At one point it seems to be defined in terms of an outreach version of the psychologist, and at another as the broker for other services. One wonders whether the author had the role explained fully to him.

## The extent of surgery

Partridge considers how much elective surgery the individual should undergo. Although once again no reference is made to the author's own circumstances, no other source or reference is quoted, and one feels that he is offering a valuable distillation of his own experiences. He introduces a concept which does not appear elsewhere in the literature -a feeling of obligation to society to proceed with a minimum acceptable level of reconstruction:

> Facial disfigurement is, above all, a social handicap, and your course of surgery to try to diminish it must at least partially respect the wishes of the wider society in which you will circulate. This may suggest that you have to fulfil certain minimum social standards when deciding on how much plastic surgery to receive - and these are not easily discovered.[10]

On the other hand, he counsels  avoidance of the need to seek perfection. This is unrealistic, and it also leads to using disfigurement as an excuse for other failings.

Nowhere in his calculation and comparison of "the benefits of further facial advances with the costs on your time and lifestyle of doing so"[11] does Partridge refer to the substantial financial costs of plastic surgery. All of his treatment was obtained in teaching hospitals within the National Health Service, and so was free at the point of use, but if the calculation is to include a social responsibility factor, and he says that it should, this cost must at least be acknowledged.


## Reconstructing your life

Part Two is concerned with the rehabilitative process:

> You are at a crossroads: in one direction lies a life of less stress but one of less excitement; in the other, the one that I hope you will choose, lies a life full of challenges, and pitfalls too. To take it, to decide to take on your face and live a full life by 'normal society' standards is difficult, but it can be done. The rest of the book is intended to help you to do it.[12]

Partridge makes a useful distinction between "personal disfigurement" and "social disfigurement"[13] - how you see yourself and your disfigurement, and how others see you. This is a useful clarification and distinction. Elsewhere too it is evident that he is drawing on others' theoretical insights within this section. References are made, direct and indirect, to Goffman. For example, he draws on his terminology, using expressions such as "discrediting".[14] He uses the concept of stigma, but qualifies Goffman's position by acknowledging that the discredited person continues to have social responsibilities, and the obligation to seek the least painful way of interacting with others pain may be sustained by the stigmatised person or by the other, and Goffman's chief emphasis is on the stigmatised person alone.

The section is a combination of very important first principles of behaviour, and of more specific hints on how to handle certain situations. Some of these latter are valuable, and they are good illustrations of the general principles; others are lacking the crispness and precision needed to put them into practice. The most powerful of the general principles is expressed in unequivocal terms:

You have lost automatic social acceptance.[15]

Consequently, the disfigured person needs to strive all of the way, and believe that he or she will achieve as much as the person without disfigurement. This will be done through recognising fully that there is a perceived differentness, and countering that differentness by complete confidence and openness. It is no longer possible for the previously reserved person to remain so - they will need to move positively to face people, explain the reasons for their different appearance, and give people the opportunity to judge them by their actions rather than by their appearance.

## Being different in public

These precepts are to be applied in a variety of situation. For example, when people are inappropriately curious (c.f. Goffman[16]), the disfigured person needs to give permission to the observer to breach accepted social boundaries, as an open response helps to make friends.[17] Where Goffman sees the intrusion as offensive, Partridge accepts that it has happened and advises making capital out of it.

This same pragmatism is evident when the question of jobs is referred to. He acknowledges that it will not always be possible to follow a career which is in the public eye,[18] but suggests that such preconceptions must be challenged appropriately.[19]

When faced with the fear or curiosity of children, the same principles apply. Society has made certain that from early years disfigurement is associated with evil,[20] but the reactions of children must be met with patience and explanation. An exception must be made in the case of older children in groups - there is little chance of winning over a gang of taunting youths, and walking away is the only valuable outcome.[21]

In contrast, some of Partridge's advice is at a higher level, and not so directly applicable. The exhortation to see the adversity as a means of enhancing family relationships,[22] for example, and needs to be broken down into its component parts before its use can become evident.

A range of resources is covered. Self-help groups are touched on, but one wonders what experience, if any, the author has had of them, as a "feel" for them is not gained.[23] While camouflage make-up is referred to,[24] curiously the Disfigurement Guidance Centre in Fife is not (apart from being mentioned in the list of useful resources at the end). Some helpful advice is given on the use of "props" such as hats, glasses and scarves; generally, they may be of temporary use, but must not become essential components of the new self-image.[25]

The need for publication is stressed, and the responsibility of everyone, including those who are disfigured, is stated. The contribution of television documentaries is acknowledged, although not always accurately, - On two occasions David Jackson is referred to as Brazilian, not Peruvian!

Partridge starts from his own experience, and from there moves to offering a framework for living for those who undergo similar experiences. In addition, he provides much material of value to therapeutic professions, in formulating methods of responding to the needs of disfigured people.


**Simon Weston**

Simon Weston's[26] experience as a Welsh Guardsman who took part in the Falklands War is told in his autobiography, "Walking Tall." He wrote about how he was injured when the landing ship Sir Galahad was bombed; he sustained severe burns to almost half of his body, and his face and hands were grossly mutilated.

## Background

Simon Weston was born and brought up in the Welsh village of Nelson, in Mid Glamorgan. The most powerful forces in his childhood were his mother (who was a district nurse in the village) and even more so his grandmother, who acted as the anchor point and support of all the family. His father is not described as influential, and his parents separated when Simon was fourteen.

As Weston was approaching school leaving age, his attitude, values and behaviour were giving his mother much cause for concern - heavy drinking, street fighting, and violent disagreements with his sister. With much pushing from his mother, Weston made application to join the army, and he was ultimately accepted by the Welsh Guards. Before this, however, he was arrested for his part in an escapade in which he and his drunken friends took a car and drove it to Cardiff. At this time he was 15 years old. He talks movingly of the shame which this brought both to himself and to his mother, and said that he felt that she would never forgive him for it.

Early days in the Welsh Guards are described in detail - the basic training, and the tours in Northern Ireland and Germany. Simon Weston became thoroughly engrossed in the army, and it became the source of his values, his friends, his social life. He absorbed all the good and the bad of army life - he had an immense pride and sense of belonging, and he also participated fully in the excesses of the social life.

Then came the South Atlantic campaign, and once more the pride and fulfilment of the professional soldier was evident. His description of the early stages of the re-taking of the Falklands indicates complete absorption and involvement in the military process.

## Becoming disfigured

Weston had already been ashore on the islands, and was being prepared for a further landing and active attack on the Argentinean position when the landing ship Sir Galahad was attacked, and he and many of his fellow soldiers were overwhelmed by a devastating fire. Like Partridge, Weston remembered every detail vividly, and the experience remained with him. It was some time before he realised how serious his condition was, and he managed these early stages through a combination of bravado and cursing. Weston was a professional soldier, with all of the bravery and bravado of which such soldiers are capable; immediately after being brought ashore at Ajax Bay he was shouting encouragement to those who were continuing the fight. At a very early stage he sought confirmation that his sexual organs were intact, saying that he would have found life difficult to continue if they had not been so.

## Reaction to disfigurement

The first time that Weston was given an indication of his mutilation was when he shouted encouragement to some paratroopers:

> We passed a group of cammed-up Paras on the way. 'Stick it to 'em for the Welsh Guards, lads,' I shouted. These were the tough, battle-hardened veterans of Goose Green, yet they looked horrified at the sight of me. A great number of us wounded were in a terrible state, shocked, burned, maimed and bleeding.[27]

The bravado continued during his emergency treatment, as he joked with the medical officer treating him as to which of them was the uglier. Little serious reference was made in the early stages to his appearance, in contrast to his overwhelming anxiety about his sex organs being intact.

One would have expected that when he first saw himself, and saw the extent of his facial injuries, Weston would have been horrified. However, he had not appreciated that his burns would leave serious and lasting disfigurement:

> I was really not conscious at this stage of how badly injured I was. Looking in the mirror, I could still say to myself, 'You don't look too bad at all, old son - once you get the scabs off, you'll be all right.'[28]

Of far more importance to him at this stage was fear of blindness, a fear which he admitted to the surgeon when reconstructive work began:

> I took a deep breath and told him about the nightmare I'd had ever since I was choppered to Ajax Bay. 'At the moment I'm petrified of going blind, absolutely petrified.'[29]

Fortunately, reconstructive surgery was completely successful in restoring the eyes to normal functioning. However, Weston was not able to escape another fear of his, the fear of pain. He is utterly honest, both in describing the actual pain, and his reactions to it:

> When it came to pain, I began to look for the easy option. Sometimes it was excruciating, climb-up-the-wall sort of pain, at other times it was simply unbearable. A sort of background burning was always there as well, as the nerve-endings grew back, but I had to learn to live with that.[30]

### Consequences of injury and disfigurement

Weston was brought back to Britain, and the slow process of reconstruction began. Early stages of work in the Queen Elizabeth Military Hospital in Woolwich are described, and a range of emotions exposed - frustration, anger, patience, and even humour (for example the irony of his face being partially reconstructed from a graft from his buttocks gave him a perverse satisfaction).

Originally, he had assumed that he would recover fully, and that he would be back to playing rugby in no time. However, although he was over-optimistic, nonetheless he wanted to be told the truth. This is broadly the same paradox described by Partridge, of finding the right balance between optimism and realism:

> She never tried to pull the wool over my eyes, even when she knew that a firm answer to my optimistic questions might throw me into a pit of depression. And she was right not to. We Welsh might suffer from verbal diarrhoea, but it means we can spot bullshit a mile off.[31]

Weston underwent numerous operations to reconstruct his face and hands. He describes the process in some detail, in non-technical language, and helps the lay person to understand the complexities of skin grafting:

> The grafts were to live on my tissue juices for the next thirty-six hours while that process was going on. Providing that the transplanted skin was kept still and in close contact with the prepared surface, there was a good chance that new vessels would grow and the graft would take. The grafted skin was

125

stitched in place to stop it skidding about when the dressing was put on.[32]

Not only was the physical process described vividly, but also Weston describes what it all felt like - the humiliation of complete physical dependency on others, the fear and loneliness of being a patient, and the wearing effect of constant pain. He obtained help in ordering his narrative for publication (from Martyn Forrester, whose exact status is not described), but the thoughts, feelings, and many of the words are clearly straight from Weston himself.

Only at this point did he admit that disfigurement bothered him:

> Somebody could have told me every day that I was going to be permanently disfigured, and I wouldn't have heard them. I didn't want to know.[33]

Simple denial was being used most effectively to make the situation tolerable.

Plastic surgery achieved much for Simon Weston, but nonetheless he was not able to continue his career in the armed forces. He had permanently sensitive hands, although they had received extensive grafts, and he was severely scarred, both from the original burns, and also from the skin donor sites all over his body. He was discharged on medical grounds, and encouraged to find an alternative, civilian, occupation. However, he was at a loss to know what, since army life was all he had known for all his adult life, and he had always assumed that his career was assured.

His reaction was to withdraw into a severe depression, drinking heavily, staying in his room and only emerging to go out at nights to drink.

Facial disfigurement was less of a problem for Weston as long as he was in a familiar setting, with familiar people. Problems were encountered when he was in a new area, or with strangers, particularly curious or hostile ones. To some extent the way was eased for him by the BBC documentaries about his experiences, but this was not always so. He was frequently stared at by strangers, particularly children:

> Sometimes on a train people would keep on and on staring, and when they looked too long I felt like jumping up and poking them in the eye. I knew very well that if I had been them I'd have stared too, because it's human nature. But I got fed up with being looked upon as a freak.[34]

126

It required courage and perseverance over a considerable time, before he felt at ease over his appearance.

## Recovery

In desperation, Weston's mother contacted his regiment, and an officer called within days to invite him to join the Guards on a rugby tour in Germany. He gained strength from the renewed association with his peers, but even more from the way in which they handled him - no allowance was made for disability, and he got no help unless he asked for it:

> I was in Germany for nearly three weeks. When I came back I was a changed person. There was this scarred boy coming back a scarred man. And it was thanks to the lads and their no-nonsense, no-pussyfooting attitude.[35]

At times this approach may seem harsh, such as the occasion when a Guardsman reproached him forcefully for not making the effort to raise his thumb to shake hands properly. However, the approach worked and Weston had reached a turning point. This was reinforced when he got home, and saw himself on the second of his T.V. documentaries, "Simon's Peace," in which he was at his most depressed and negative.

A range of opportunities were then offered to him, which he used to the full - travel to the Guards Association in New Zealand and Australia, participation in Operation Raleigh, and learning to fly. Weston had caught the attention of influential people - it was the Prince of Wales who nominated him for Operation Raleigh.

He was sponsored on his flying course by King Hussein of Jordan, and it was when the king was visiting the flying school at Kidlington that Weston reached another significant point in his recovery. Suddenly, as he was recounting his experiences over lunch to King Hussein, he became aware that he did not want to talk about it any more - he wanted to move on, and give the stage to someone else:

> It seemed that I always got pushed to the forefront, but now I suddenly felt that it was someone else's turn.
>
> ...If I am entering a new phase of my life, I thought, one in which memories of the Falklands will play a progressively

smaller and smaller role, then perhaps I should commit those memories to paper before they fade for ever.[36]

Simon Weston overcame major physical and emotional obstacles partly by means of his nerve and courage, but also by finding another purpose for living when being a soldier was no longer open to him. He established a charity, Weston Spirit, whose aim was to instill in young people living in depressed cities in Britain an enthusiasm to help others in their communities. This was to be achieved by the provision of residential training courses in the country.

> .... a balanced programme of action and reflection. The courses would serve as a beginning, not as an end in themselves. Participants would be supported on their return home in the development of local enterprise projects, which would identify needs and seek solutions.[37]

So Weston found meaning and purpose in his life by helping others - as in their own ways did Trust, Piff and Partridge. Many of those who helped him were soldiers - officers and members of his regiment in the early days, but long afterwards he continued to have a rapport with soldiers and ex-soldiers - his close colleague in the establishment of the trust, Paul Oginsky, was a member of the TA Parachute Regiment. But what also helped him was his own sense of the wastefulness of inertia and loss of motivation. What he had almost lost himself was so precious that he wanted to see it restored in others.

### Doreen Trust

By way of contrast, it is worth mentioning another author whose original inspiration came from her own disfigurement. However, she does not write to describe this experience. Rather, she speaks from the position of teacher and adviser. Doreen Trust,[38] Director of the Disfigurement Guidance Centre in Cupar, Fife, has a congenital disfigurement - a facial port-wine stain. She is a professional person (a trained teacher), and her husband, who works with her at the Centre, is an artist. In addition, however, she has become a professional helper of others in conditions to which she relates by virtue of her own situation.

"Overcoming Disfigurement" describes early references to disfigurement, and provides background material about those who have helped disfigured people. However, the purpose of the book is principally to advise and encourage families who have a member with a disfigurement. It does not describe the experience of the individual who has become or who is disfigured. It is simply mentioned here because of the author's disfigurement; it would seem probable that this was her motivation and inspiration for undertaking this work, but this is never stated.

Much of this book is positive, stimulating and comforting; it is aimed at the parents of disfigured children, but a great deal of it could be applied to bringing up any child. One therefore feels that it is not quite as focused as it might be. This is remarkable, considering the extent of experience of the author, both personal and professional.

## Christine Piff

The final book reviewed in this chapter is also written by a woman, and one whose experience is most material to the present study. Christine Piff[39] was thirty-five, married with three children, when she was diagnosed as having facial cancer. She had previously been very healthy, and led an active life as a parent, wife and nursery nurse. Her book makes it clear that she was (and is) a most fulfilled person, whose family life was secure and firm. She was determined, a fighter, and one who appreciated the value of life and family relationships. She was passionately fond of children:

> My whole life, it seemed, revolved around children, for as a qualified Nursery Nurse I also spent every morning at a local play school. This didn't interfere with my husband or my children and it satisfied a need in me to be with the people I like best: children.[40]

## Illness and treatment

Shortly before Christmas 1986, Christine began to suffer severe facial pain. A few weeks into the New Year, she was admitted to hospital for an exploratory operation, which revealed a tumour in her sinus. This was treated first by radiotherapy, and subsequently by surgery.

Following radiotherapy and surgery, which involved the excision of her palate, Christine was devastated to learn that malignant cells were still present, and she had to go to London for more radical surgery.

Hitherto she had preserved much of her outward facial appearance, and contrary to expectations she had retained the sight in her left eye. Now she lost her eye, the orbit which retains the eye, and much of her left cheek. So not only did she have to face the possibility of further illness and death, but she was also severely disfigured.

Christine Piff has survived, and has established a most influential support group for people with facial disfigurement, described in the chapter on mutual help. Her path to survival has many lessons for professionals, others with facial cancer and other forms of facial disfigurement, and for their families and friends.


## Reactions to illness and disfigurement

At every stage of being told bad news, Christine was simply overwhelmed by distress. She was shocked, and deeply upset. The causes were two-fold - the first was fear of death:

> The thought of me dying and leaving him and the children on their own was more than I could bear.[41]

She had a very full life, principally taken up by her family - immediate and extended - and by working with children, and she had a lot to lose. More than that, she could not bear the thought of her family having to do without her:

> The thought of not sharing the rest of his life with him was worse than any physical torture. Not to be with the children any more, not to be there to help Claire grow into a woman, to share her joys and her sorrows. Matthew - how would he take my dying?...Little Dominic... he was the youngest, would it be easier for him or not?[42]

Generally, she reacted as people do react to loss, including feelings of disbelief and denial. In addition, she found herself unable to absorb things which professionals were telling her. For example, prior to the first operation, two professionals made it clear to her that the excision of her palate would present her with speech problems. She remembered this afterwards, but did not absorb it at the time, and was surprised:

> The sounds didn't come out the way I wanted and my voice

was totally unfamiliar. This was obviously due to the obturator in my mouth. I remembered what Mr. Issa had said about not being able to speak without it.[43]

Other differences and changes were understated by professionals, and she had to find out for herself.

From time to time during the period of treatment and recovery, Christine was touchy, and inclined to bad temper. That she had a patient and even-tempered partner must have been a great help when she flung hairbrushes and saucepans around. Her husband Chris was her antithesis; he felt her illness and the treatment process acutely, but in day to day life he was very hard to ruffle. When Christine had been particularly outrageous one day, his comment to the children was

Nothing your mother does could surprise me.[44]

When treatment was finally over, and the rehabilitation phase was reached, Christine was left with a large cavity where her eye and its orbit had been, and part of her cheek had been removed. This had to be filled by an artificial structure, a prosthesis. This gave her face its normal contour, but the fluctuations of colour and texture of the face cannot be reproduced exactly, and it was not possible to disguise completely the joint between the real and artificial part, or the immobile false eye. Although the prosthesis was preferable to wearing an eye patch, she was still lacking in confidence when she wished to go outside and face strangers. With friends and relatives she was more comfortable - indeed her children had told all their school friends and they wanted to come round to have a look. She was happy to explain to children how the prosthesis worked (in later years she began to carry a spare around with her to show children), but she never showed the cavity to anyone except clinical staff. Her husband and children never saw it. She herself was ill-prepared for seeing it, and was devastated when she caught sight of herself in a mirror in the hospital, and she never wished others to have to handle the feelings involved. This relates to James Partidge's view of the disfigured person's social responsibility to achieve a degree of normality in order not to inflict unacceptable appearance on others.


## Consequences of illness and disfigurement

Most of the changes in Christine Piff's life were more directly related

131

to the consequences of treatment than to the illness itself. Treatment was successful; she sustained a life-threatening illness and with the removal of the malignant tissue the immediate threat receded. So the main consequence of the illness itself was the fear of dying, and this remained. She also suffered substantial weight loss, but this was due to a large extent to not being able to eat during the course of treatment.

Christine was warned of the side effects of radiotherapy - sickness and hair loss, and she was in part prepared, but she was not ready for the extent of the hair loss, and she was devastated:

> By the time I had combed it all, the hair was piled in mounds around my shoulders....I couldn't contain myself any longer, the deep grief I felt exploded inside me and I cried and cried, inconsolable.[45]

This was because of the destruction of tissue by the radiotherapy. Other problems were related directly to surgery. In particular, because part of her mouth had been removed, Christine found eating and speaking very difficult. She had to learn how to speak again, with part of the roof of her mouth replaced by an artificial obturator. Eating was similarly a skill which she had to acquire over again, and initially, eating solids was virtually impossible. This contributed to her loss of weight.

Appearance itself was a problem. It was some time before she was used to people staring, and it was her own view of herself which had to gain strength before she could tolerate others looking at her. She was terrified of her family's reactions, and indeed they never actually saw her without either a dressing or prosthesis.

The more profound effects on the family are described. In particular, her older son Matthew was severely troubled by the experience, and only gradually overcame it. He became withdrawn and tearful, ran away from school, and ceased to have his previous enthusiasm for life. It was literally years before he began to be convinced that he was not going to lose his mother through death.

A nursery nurse by profession, Christine was particularly troubled that her illness and treatment meant that she could no longer work in the playgroup. Subsequently, she filled her days with activity and purpose, but working with children had been much of her reason for being, and so she sustained a deep loss when she was no longer able to do so.

## Comments on professional intervention

Generally, professionals are referred to warmly and with gratitude. Two professions in particular are acknowledged for their sympathy and understanding attitude. First, nurses are praised for the way in which they helped Christine through difficult times, encouraging and cajoling her, and showing that they understood the need for personal touches (such as putting her own clothes on her as soon as possible after surgery). There are exceptions - particularly the plastic surgery sister who was asked to remove her stitches, and who vented all her frustrations on the sister from Christine's ward, in front of Christine:

> The outburst that followed amazed me. The gist of it was that nobody ever told her anything, she wasn't going to do it, she was far too busy with her patients, it just couldn't be done and a few more exasperated sentences.[46]

The second professional who received praise was the maxillo-facial technician (It was a maxillo-facial technician who first drew to the attention of the present author the social and emotional needs of disfigured people). The way in which they were completely accepting of her mutilated appearance was valued, and the skill and artistry with which they overcame technical problems was praised. Typically, the technician develops a close working relationship with the patient, and this continues to be so in Christine's case:

> Not only is he talented and blessed with a rare gift but he is also aware of the deep emotional struggle his patients are going through. He has the capacity of being able to fill them with confidence and total trust in what he is doing.[47]

Not all professional responses were perfect. Some professionals, particularly the surgeons, were quite low-key and matter of fact, and their detachment caused some surprise. She described how her surgeon had reacted dispassionately when she complained of noises in the ear:

> Oh yes, there's a name for noises in the ear, he said. It has been known to drive people mad. I sat there looking at Mr. Wallace, and I wanted to laugh. It was rather like a mechanic telling you your engine is loose, but not to worry, if it fell out you might crash, although then again you might not.[48]

133

She also felt that some things which were going to happen to her were under-described, but equally she acknowledged that there were times when she could not absorb what she was being told. Presumably the clinicians were making constant calculations about how much information to transmit at any one time. Partridge said that the truth must be filtered in order to keep the patient positive. To this is now added the suggestion that the clinician must present the truth in manageable amounts.

### Recovery

Christine Piff demonstrated nerve and courage in her recovery from cancer. The part played by her attitude in overcoming illness cannot be quantified, but it must be recognised as substantial:

> Reality suddenly came back and kicked me hard in the stomach. 'Oh my God!' I flung myself on to the bed and wept. Then, equally quickly, 'Christine' took over again, confident and determined. I dried my eyes and took stock of myself. 'So, I have cancer. Right. Well, I'll treat it like 'flu. We'll treat it and get over it.'[49]

An element in this positive attitude was her humour. She and her family could frequently find a funny side to an incident or a situation, which otherwise would be quite depressing. Her attempts at using a monocle to read is one situation. Another was her reaction to her hair growing back curly following its loss through radiation, when she claimed that "cancer gives you curls." On occasions some might find her humour inappropriate or jarring:

> When I couldn't stand it any longer, I said, 'Looking at the funny pictures?'

> On reflection it was a stupid thing to say, and Dr. Strickland must have thought so too. He retorted, 'Not so funny, my dear. In fact, very serious ones'.[50]

However, as a means of facing intolerable pain and worry, her humour was successful. Like much humour, it appears harsh when examined out of context.

The other major resource which enabled recovery and rehabilitation was Christine's family. They contributed in two ways. First, she received constant encouragement and positive stimulus from them. From her husband she received patience, understanding and much practical help. From her children she was constantly reassured that it was important to get better and quickly. Second, she knew that she was needed, and having important people in her life who needed her meant that she could not give up.

The other stimulus to survive and keep living is described in Chapter Six, the establishment of the group Let's Face It. The group absorbs much time and energy, and is a further illustration of the strong hold which this remarkable woman has on life and people.

### Conclusions

1.  How much reconstructive surgery the individual should undergo is hard to say; the calculation has many components, including the stamina of the patient, and what level of restoration makes them acceptable to themselves. It is also suggested that the disfigured person should try to make themselves look acceptable to others.

2.  The surgeon needs to be able to talk to patients, explaining their condition, the proposed treatment, and the likely consequences.

3.  The question of honesty to the patient is discussed, but all three authors feel that it is important for information-giving to be measured and timed.

4.  The process of surgery is referred to in detail by all three authors. Partridge said that the patient should acquire fluency with medical terminology. Weston's and Christine Piff's jargon-free descriptions would suggest that this is not necessary.

5.  The patient needs to keep some control over his situation. All three main authors reviewed in this chapter were strong-minded people, for whom this might not be a problem. Others might find it more difficult to feel powerful in the patient role.

6.  The importance of a range of professionals is emphasised, in

addition to surgeons and nurses. The roles of psychologist, social worker and maxillo-facial technician are discussed.

7. The disfigured person must develop strategies for handling public reaction. While the reactions of children may be most probing, children may also be the most refreshing, ingenuous and accepting.

8. The potential for depression and giving up is considerable, and the pressures strong - length of treatment, pain, changed appearance, changed lifestyle. Humour helped some. Partridge survived by making rational sense of the process. All three became in some way public figures.

9. For all the authors the experience of disfigurement was a major upheaval in their lives, but one which each of them turned to advantage and enrichment.

10. Disfigurement is loss - loss of face, health, mobility, acceptance and ease in relationships, and job. The individual handles the stages of recovery from this loss in just the same way as they would deal with any other serious loss, such as a bereavement.

**Notes**

1. Howell, M. and Ford, P., 1980, *The True History of the Elephant Man,* Allison and Busby, London.
2. Partridge, J., 1990, *Changing Faces - The Challenge of Facial Disfigurement,* Penguin, Harmondsworth.
3. op. cit., biographical note.
4. op. cit., p. 22.
5. op. cit., p. 40.
6. op. cit., p. 55.
7. op. cit., p. 38.
8. op. cit., p. 79.
9. op. cit., p. 62.
10. op. cit., p. 48.
11. op. cit., p. 50.
12. op. cit., p. 33.
13. op. cit., p. 60.

14. op. cit., p. 122.
15. op. cit., p. 67.
16. Goffman, E., 1964, *Stigma*, Penguin, Harmondsworth.
17. Partridge, op. cit., p. 91.
18. op. cit., p. 70.
19. op. cit., p. 126.
20. op. cit., p. 100.
21. op. cit., p. 101.
22. op. cit., p. 112.
23. op. cit., p. 84.
24. op. cit., p. 79.
25. op. cit., p. 105.
26. Weston, S., 1989, *Walking Tall*, Bloomsbury, London.
27. op. cit., p. 157.
28. op. cit., p. 166.
29. op. cit., p. 186.
30. op. cit., p. 175.
32. op. cit., p. 185.
32. op. cit., p. 187.
33. op. cit., p. 189.
34. op. cit., p. 199.
35. op. cit., p. 208.
36. op. cit., p. 239.
37. op. cit., p. 226.
38. Trust, D.S., 1986 *Overcoming Disfigurement: defeating the problems - physical, social and emotional*, Thorsons, Wellingborough.
39. Piff, C., 1985, *Let's Face It*, Victor Gollancz, London.
40. op. cit., p. 10.
41. op. cit., p. 68.
42. ibid.
43. op. cit., p. 46.
44. op. cit., p. 111.
45. op. cit., p. 62.
46. op. cit., p. 52.
47. op. cit., p. 124.
48. op. cit., p. 99.
49. op. cit., p. 14.
50. op. cit., p. 15.

# PART II
# HELPING DISFIGURED PEOPLE

# 5 Mutual help groups

Voluntary groups have emerged since the beginning of World War II, in the United Kingdom and elsewhere, composed almost entirely of disfigured people. In all, three such groups have been identified, and the occasions for them coming into being, and the purposes for their continued existence, vary. This chapter describes the origins of these groups, the purposes for which they were established and are maintained, and the activities which they undertake. The nature of the relationship between members is examined, in order to understand the value of the groups. An attempt is made, using facial disfigurement groups as an illustration, to establish how far people with similar severe social needs can be of help to each other.

The first group is a highly specialised one known as the Guinea Pig Club, composed almost entirely of R.A.F. personnel who suffered burns during World War II. The second is the most widespread mutual help group for people with a facial disfigurement in the U.K., Let's Face It. This was approached from two perspectives; the national organiser and founder was interviewed, and then the organiser of a local group, in order to see whether there was any difference in their beliefs and practices. Finally, the issues were discussed with the staff of the Disfigurement Guidance Centre in Fife. This is not a mutual help group, but the staff have organised such groups in the past, and have very strong beliefs and feelings about them. Leaders of these groups were interviewed; their responses, which provided material for this chapter, are summarised below in Table 6.1. Groups exist in other countries which have similarities to the British groups - Les Gueules Cassees in France, Let's Face It in the U.S.A., and About Face in Ontario. These were not included in the analysis, although some literature has been received from the U.S.A. branch of Let's Face It.

## The Guinea Pig Club

The Guinea Pig Club was established in July 1941, by the men of the R.A.F., Commonwealth and allied air forces who were burned or otherwise mutilated during the Battle of Britain. Initially, it was formed to perpetuate the comradeship formed at the Queen Victoria Hospital, East Grinstead. Although it was established as something of a joke by some of the patients of Ward III, the underlying need was serious. The original intention, according to its founders, was to meet every year for the purpose of "consuming large quantities of beer in each others' company." To be more serious, it was felt by these men that they needed to band together in order to survive the physical and emotional hardships which they could expect to face. In this they were strongly encouraged by their surgeon, (later Sir) Archibald McIndoe:

> Stick together and no power on earth can break you. Fall apart and you've had it.

## Background - McIndoe and East Grinstead

Just before the Second World War, in preparation for the anticipated numbers of burn injuries which would arise from war in the air, the Royal Air Force designated the Queen Victoria Hospital, East Grinstead, as a special Plastic and Reconstructive Surgery Unit; it was particularly intended for airmen who might sustain the severe burns associated with flying, due especially to the volatility of aviation fuel. During the early months of the war, only a handful of patients were treated, but when the Battle of Britain began, large numbers of R.A.F. staff had cause to be taken to Ward III at East Grinstead. By the end of the war, 647 air force personnel had been treated at the hospital. In addition, some naval and army personnel were also treated. The injuries and burns which the patients suffered brought new challenges to the surgical staff. Archie McIndoe was invited to be consultant in charge of the unit; he agreed, and in the course of the war not only did he pioneer new techniques in reconstructive surgery; he also inspired his patients to adopt positive attitudes which vastly assisted their recovery and rehabilitation.

Many of the patients had similar patterns of injuries, which came to be known as "standard Hurricane burns" - severe burns to the legs, forearms and face, including the eyelids. New techniques of grafting and constructing pedicles were put to the test. Therapeutic aids, such

142

as bathing in saline solution, were developed, and older techniques, such as the application of tannic acid, were discredited.

In addition to the skills as a plastic surgeon which McIndoe undoubtedly had, his success with the patients of his ward was also due to a large extent to the positive attitude which he engendered in them. He was utterly open with them about their injuries, their appearance, and their chances of successful rehabilitation. The patients concerned were not strangers to facing unpalatable truths; they reacted positively to his invitation to come to the operating theatre to observe procedures being carried out on their colleagues which they themselves were about to undergo.

A greater freedom and tolerance of patients was allowed on the ward than was usual at that time. Airmen who were ambulant would visit local pubs, often pushing their less mobile colleagues. Discipline was less exacting on the ward than was then normally accepted. Initially this met with objections from other hospital staff, but these ceased when it became clear that McIndoe's patients had a faster recovery rate than patients elsewhere in the hospital. Determination characterised the atmosphere of the unit - McIndoe was determined to make his patients whole, and they were determined to get back to fight again; about one third did so, and several were injured again and returned to East Grinstead.

## The origins of the Club

The Guinea Pig Club was founded, in July, 1941, by several of the patients of Ward III, initially in order to perpetuate the comradeship which had been engendered by their shared experience of mutilation, treatment and recovery at East Grinstead. The members agreed to meet annually in order to maintain contact and recall the comradeship. The name came about through a wry conversation a few days earlier between two of the patients, when they summed up their current status by observing that they were McIndoe's guinea pigs.

## The welfare element of the Club

Initially, reunion was the principal theme, but by the end of the war it had become evident that many of the Guinea Pigs were to have serious problems in re-integrating into civilian life, because of disability, sensory loss, problems arising from disfigurement, and emotional reactions to their wartime experiences. At the annual dinner a surgeon was always in attendance to advise on clinical matters, and later a welfare service was also made available. This continued as a permanent feature in the post-war years, but it was not sufficient to respond to the day-to-day problems experienced by members. Consequently, a full-time welfare element was established, and this continues to the present day. The service is funded by the R.A.F. Benevolent Fund, and aims to alleviate hardship of any kind for members of the club. Unsolicited donations are also received from elsewhere, but no fundraising is required.

Many members of the club are resistant to the notion of charity, and it is stressed that there is no suggestion of getting something for nothing with no effort of one's own; charity is seen by the Guinea Pigs as "solving someone else's problems by involving oneself." Typically, the assistance given is financial - for example, to assist a member to begin his own business. In one instance this was done for an ex-airman who was having difficulty in accepting the constraints of time-keeping and organisational requirements; the club responded by helping him become his own boss.

Three precepts are kept in mind by the officers of the club who are responsible for welfare. The first is to keep in mind constantly the fact that many of the members are likely to react badly to stress, having been subjected to extreme stresses during the conflict. Maximum effort should be put into assisting them when this stress is evident.

Secondly, the club believes that welfare effort should be channelled towards helping establish a member in the community, rather than simply providing subsistence. To provide direct income would, in their eyes, sap initiative.

Finally, the most tragic thought for members of the club is that they should be forgotten, by their colleagues, or by their country. They will remain sensitive to this possibility, and will resent any incident or set of circumstances which reinforces this idea.


## The effectiveness of the Club

Almost all of the members of the Guinea Pig Club were fully rehabilitated after the war, either back to the armed services or into civilian occupations. The initial purpose of the club, the perpetuation of comradeship which war, fighting together and recovering from injuries together had inspired, was achieved, and continues to be achieved. This is through the annual reunion weekend and through other contact which individual members have with each other.

As the members have aged, so their dependency needs have increased. Their physical ageing processes have been aggravated by the special problems which scarred tissue presents, and other disabilities which they have lived with over the last forty-five or fifty years. Now, they are all of retirement age or over, and survivors are likely to become even more dependent, on their families, their colleagues, and on professionals. In these circumstances, effective welfare is even more vital, and the club acknowledges this by stepping up their attention to their members' dependency needs.

The Guinea Pig Club was a special situation, in which the comradeship of the war, and the fellowship of being treated in the same unit by pioneer methods, were at least as important as the issue of disfigurement. Members of the club have been able to make use of the disadvantage by making of it a virtue - by defining themselves as an exclusive group, and making access to their privileges unattainable for those who have not experienced the same adversities and set-backs. In a similar way, Simon Weston, who was severely burned in active service on the Sir Galahad during the Falklands conflict (BBC, April 1989), made use of the renown which it brought him to help establish his venture trust Weston Spirit. Other groups for people with a facial disfigurement lack such an association with heroism and military comradeship. Do they have the same cohesiveness, success and ability to meet the needs of their members through mutual dependence and giving? The best-established group for disfigured people in general in the U.K. is Let's Face It, a national network of support systems established by Christine Piff in 1984.

**Let's Face It**

Christine Piff established Let's Face It, a support network for people with facial disfigurements, in 1984. In that year, Channel Four Television made a programme describing the problems faced by disfigured people, and featuring Christine. Because of the high level of interest expressed in the programme, and because of the number of people with problems who made contact with her as a direct result of it, she decided that there was a need to establish an organisation to meet their needs. The group would have two aims. The most important was to act as special friends to each other; repeatedly the statement is made by Christine that no one can understand the problems of disfigurement except those who are themselves disfigured. The friends would therefore be in a unique position in relation to each other, meeting needs which no one else, not even other family members, could do.

Secondly, Let's Face It aims to raise awareness amongst health care professionals about the problems encountered by disfigured people, and improve their sensitivity to their patients. The group recognises and is grateful for the skills of all professionals - surgeons, radiotherapists, anaesthetists, nurses, maxillo-facial technicians, occupational therapists and social workers - but asks them to consider their work in a broader context. When the highly-skilled clinical work has been carried out, how do the results get communicated to patients and their families, and what is life like ever after.

Christine Piff's understanding of the problems of disfigured people began with her own experience of having facial cancer, and all that followed from this. Her personal story is told in her first book, Let's Face It,[1] an intimate account of diagnosis, surgery and follow-up monitoring of her condition; subsequently, she suffered a recurrence, and had to undergo substantial resection of the face.

These experiences were devastating. Christine Piff recounts a number of situations which she faced with professionals, all of which demonstrated that they had failed to see things from her point of view - understanding of the diagnosis, recognising fully the nature and extent of the surgery, what her face would look like after surgery, what reaction people had to seeing her face after it had been substantially mutilated (albeit to save her life). She felt that people avoided her, finding her appearance too painful for them to tolerate. She too reacted badly to it, and despite the strong support of her husband and family felt quite alone. No one saw it as important that she should have someone with her when she first looked in the mirror, or when she thought for days on how to reconstruct her life. It was insights like this that caused her to believe that only other disfigured people could fully appreciate what others in her situation were going through. To ensure that this understanding, compassion and backing were provided, she established the network.


## Organisation

Let's Face It exists in the first instance for people who have suffered from any form of facial disfigurement - whether they were born with it, or acquired it through burns, other accidents, or through cancer. It also extends to the families of disfigured people, and literally anyone else with an interest or concern, including interested professionals who are involved in the healing and recovery process.

Membership of the network is extensive. There are some one thousand members, principally in the United Kingdom, the United States and South Africa. Membership is continuing to expand, particularly in the United States, where a separate structure has been established, with the approval and assistance of the original British organisation.

In fact, organisation within the original U.K. network is minimal; there are few attributes of the formal bureaucracy about Let's Face It. Informality has been a deliberate style, maintained from the outset by the founder. There is no board of directors (although the American group has them), no elaborate charter, no salaried officers, no registered office, and no extensive decision-making process. Funding is restricted to what is required for immediate campaigning purposes - travelling expenses, postage and other communication. Most of the campaigning is carried out by Christine Piff herself, and she has fostered this lean approach, spending donated money sparingly, and almost resenting any acquisition which detracts from the simplicity and directness of her message. She regards her electric typewriter almost as a luxury, while many other organisations of similar dimensions have moved on to word processors, computers and fax machines. On this typewriter she writes some one hundred individual personal letters each week to her friends in the network.

However, accounting is scrupulous, and the administration is meticulous. Both systems are kept to a necessary minimum simply in order to devote all possible energy to the maintenance of personal contact with members.

In addition to keeping in contact with individuals by letter, Christine Piff's activities include maintaining telephone links with persons in distress who need more extensive counselling than writing can provide. She offers advice on how to communicate with surgeons and physicians, how to approach discussions with dieticians, speech therapists and other professionals, and helps people to contact maxillo-facial technicians. She visits people in hospital and counsels families on managing the stresses caused by one of their members having a disfigurement. She also organises group meetings locally, establishes groups in other parts of the country, and offers social events (such as garden parties) to keep people in touch with each other and to raise funds for necessary expenses.

Campaigning on a wider basis has included lectures to professionals all over the country. Some of these contacts have contributed to the foundation of support groups, though in some instances Christine has met with a stone wall response from professionals. She has also made a second television programme, further highlighting issues of disfigurement. She has written articles, is writing a second book, and has commissioned a book for children, raising their awareness of disfigurement issues. By means of a printed newsletter she maintains quarterly contact with all her contacts, who are always described as her friends.

## Aims

The making of special friendships is the principal aim of the network. Based on the belief that disfigured people require a depth of understanding which can only be obtained from each other, it includes anyone at all for whom disfigurement is an issue, as Christine says in her promotional leaflet:

> From children born with disfigurement, burns, to cancer patients, Bell's Palsy, road accidents, teenagers with acne, women with facial hair. Young people who just feel ugly and need a friend who understands.

If members wish, they can participate in a local group, but only if they choose to:

> Everyone is different, and no pressure is put on friends to attend meetings or make any commitment. Friends take out of Let's Face It what they need at their 'special time'.

For many, however, the principal source of help and friendship is the founder herself:

> I am available seven days a week, twenty-four hours a day. I write approximately one hundred letters a week to friends. Friends expect to be able to share their worries and fears with someone else who has been 'there' giving hope and encouragement.

This is no doubt a profound source of relief and assistance to the individual; it must also be seen in terms of what it does to the one person who gives so much, and how long and how widely such an approach to helping and giving can be maintained. Roles and relationships between members of mutual help groups will be discussed below.

## Influencing professional attitudes

A further purpose for the establishment of Let's Face It was to sensitise professionals to the needs of disfigured people. In order to achieve this, Christine Piff writes to surgeons, technicians, occupational therapists, speech therapists, physiotherapists, social workers - anyone who will listen to her, repeating her message that professionals must hear what patients are saying to them. She gives lectures to professionals, often in quite daunting circumstances. The present writer has heard her speak at the Royal College of Psychiatrists, and in a Nurse Education Lecture Hall, and although she expresses diffidence, she makes her points forcibly to the professional audience. She also influences local practice by enlisting the support of professionals to establish local network groups, and her constant theme is that "we must get the professionals on our side." The evidence is growing in the literature that surgeons acknowledge that their work is only the beginning of rehabilitation. In conversation with surgeons the present author has noted some shift of emphasis; there is also some distance to travel in many instances, underlining the continued need for Let's Face It to campaign.

## Leadership of the organisation

Christine Piff occupies a special place in the group of friends; she is not simply another friend: she controls the direction and ethos of the network, she controls the spending of a national budget (however small), and she is the principal campaigner. She links with established groups throughout the country, and she works to set up new local groups. She manages and largely writes the newsletter of the network three times a year. She gives a lot of herself to members, is constantly available, and it would seem that for her the giving is sufficient reward in itself. She is a strong and determined character, giving to members in a way that she is not likely to receive from them. She is also something of a charismatic leader, sending messages of encouragement, in the newsletter and elsewhere, and keeping members up to date with her own family news, all of which is welcomed by the members. Christine Piff began the network, and it is not likely to have existed without her. She is, however, confident that it could now go on of its own momentum, even if she were no longer to be with it. When interviewed for this research she claimed that "I didn't start the Network - it started me." She felt that the need set the process going, and was resistant to the suggestion that she might have some special or exceptional quality which accounted for its success. She is fully aware of the possibility of her own death, and spends a lot of time wondering what would happen to her friends. She is confident that if she was no longer able to take a lead someone else would make themselves available and perpetuate the work. This confidence and simple trust characterises her overall approach, together with her determination not to acknowledge obstacles - "My attitude has made Let's Face It what it is."

## Local groups

A major element of Christine Piff's work has been to establish self-run groups in regional centres for those members of the network who find it helpful to have personal, face-to-face contact with each other; groups are now well- established in ten cities, with more beginning all the time. Without exception they are conducted on hospital premises. This is deliberate, based on the belief that all participants are familiar with hospitals, and find them safe places. Frequently the founder talks about the problems encountered by people who have got to grips with their illness and disfigurement in themselves, but then have to confront the wider world outside hospital - this is what presents them with difficulties, in contrast to people who have never suffered any serious or chronic illness which has required frequent hospital attendance, who often feel unsafe inside a hospital. It has been Christine's practice to gain the support of local relevant professionals in the establishment of the groups, and indeed not to proceed until she has done so. In almost every instance the contact person or facilitator is a professional - typically a nursing sister, an occupational therapist or a physiotherapist. Such a group was established in Leeds at the General Infirmary in July 1986. This group is described in detail in order to assess how similar such a group is to the original network pioneered by Christine Piff, and to identify what original or different characteristics it has. The group was set up by an occupational therapist, a speech therapist, and an ex-patient. The occupational therapist, when interviewed for this study, explained that she had seen the need for people to speak to others who had a similar problem. After working on a burns unit where an informal support group worked, she had become convinced of the advantages of such an arrangement. She had also come to realize the need to educate others on the subject of disfigurement, and to increase public awareness of the subject. The group was therefore set up, with the following specific aims:

- to provide support to those who are disfigured and their families and friends, by open meetings and telephone and postal contact;

- to provide advice and up-to-date information on issues to do with disfigurement (for example, camouflage make-up);

- to provide social functions;

- to raise funds to cover costs or for specific purposes; (for example, research projects);

- to educate the public, particularly through the media on issues of disfigurement.

The group exists for "anyone who feels that their quality of life is marred by facial problems, whatever they may be". A number of members with disfiguring conditions have responded to posters in the hospital, after attending the occupational therapist as patients. Their ages range from 20 to 65 years, and at present some 15 to 20 people attend the meetings, although the mailing list includes about 40 people. Most of the currently active members are people who have finished their treatment at the hospital. As with the national Let's Face It network, no particular type of disfigurement predominates; a range of problems and needs is addressed.

The group has distinct leaders, no matter how much attempts are made to delegate responsibilities. The position of one of the leaders in the hospital, Head Occupational Therapist, influences the way in which she is viewed by members; she is in a position of authority within the hospital, and has access to resources which the members need, individually and collectively - other professionals (as therapists and as speakers at the meetings), rooms for meetings, publicity facilities. The same applies to the speech therapist; the third leader, a former patient, is an articulate, educated person, who, like Christine Piff, is well able to hold her own and not be over-awed by the presence of professionals. Meetings take place monthly, and vary from a speaker meeting to business meetings and social events. Additional group discussions are also arranged, as well as one-to-one counselling by the professional group leaders, and telephone or letter linking for individual support. Not all members attend every month - some attend regularly, and some attend just enough to keep in contact.

In the initial phase, some members felt that they had to be constantly discussing issues of disfigurement, actively helping someone in distress, at every meeting. In fact, a wide range of people with different needs participate, and it is difficult to meet everyone's needs all the time. Not everyone could stand the intensity of focusing on disfigurement at every meeting. At a general level, several members wanted to achieve a sense of purpose - to turn their experience of injuries, problems and disease into something positive. In addition, all who came showed that they valued the meetings, and set much store by them. There was great distress if some members stopped coming; those remaining felt that they were failing, and they constantly re-assess the objectives and activities of the group. Two reasons often arise for not attending: the first is geographical - the members travel a great distance, for treatment, and for attendance at the group meetings, and regular attendance is physically difficult. The second reason is that, despite what has been said about hospital being a safe place, home is safer still, and some people are frightened of leaving that safety more than is absolutely necessary. Those who do take great comfort from meeting others who have made similar efforts.

There is a degree of structure to the organisation of the group - there is a secretary and a treasurer, minutes are maintained, and correspondence noted at each meeting. The group is self-governing, but hopes shortly to become a self- governing sub-group of the Leeds Foundation for Dermatological Research. This can be a problem, according to the leader:

> Leaders of the group can become over-burdened with organisation and need to look at delegation, but members like to have a 'leader' - especially a professional.

The presence of people of varied experiences, qualifications, skills and status within the group seems to have had the effect of making it slightly hierarchical, although the activities are conducted in a most informal manner. Some people are better than others at getting things going, and some prefer to be helped and led. To this extent the group is at times one of mutual interest rather than of mutual help. As with the welfare element of the Guinea Pig Club, some help and some are helped; the mutuality in that instance lay in the preparedness of all members to help if called upon. In the case of Leeds Let's Face It this does not appear so evident; the members do express concern for each other, but most of the individual support seems to be given by the group leaders.

Despite this, it must be emphasised that there is mutuality in the eyes of the members and the principal way in which it is expressed is by acceptance:

> When it all first started I quite agreed with Christine when she said that you'd never get a room full of people with unusual faces all together. But even Christine now admits she was wrong about that, and how glad I am that she was wrong....if we want others to accept us as we are, with our different types of face, we have to be prepared to accept the different types of people who make up our Network....With our different types of faces we are all vulnerable; we are special people.[2]

However much the members of the Leeds group lean on their leaders, they all regard each other as special, and in that lies the strength which they give to each other.

### Let's Face It in the United States

Let's Face It has also spread to the United States, on the initiative of its founder, Christine Piff. It has a more organisational focus than its British counter-part, with a board of directors, substantial grant aid from a large company, a computer-based record of members. It still has a very personal approach to providing support to members of the network, and this personal approach is led by its chairperson, Betsy Wilson. It produces a quarterly newsletter as the principal means of keeping in touch, but the same informal contacts and meetings of local groups also occur.

### The Disfigurement Guidance Centre

So far groups have been described whose leaders feel that there is value and advantage in those with similar problems being in contact with and drawing strength from each other. A dissenting voice in the positive rating of mutual help groups is the Disfigurement Guidance Centre in Cupar, Fife. This is run by Doreen Trust and her husband Peter. Together they provide a range of services for people for whom disfigurement is an issue. These include counselling of individuals, advice and guidance on camouflage make-up, education programmes in schools, lectures on attitudes to disfigurement, and drama as a means of attitude change. Although the location in Fife might be seen by many to be remote, the centre has contact with people all over the United Kingdom, many of whom attend the Centre personally. It distributes a newsletter, and its director, Doreen Trust, conducts extensive correspondence and provides telephone contact with those in need of counselling and support. The centre is maintained by grants (for example from Fife Regional Council) and voluntary contributions.

The Trusts have experimented with a variety of approaches to helping people with disfigurement, and their experience goes back almost twenty years. They have provided N.H.S. counselling and make-up advice sessions, they have travelled the country raising awareness over issues of disfigurement, and they have participated in the Manpower Services Commission training scheme for young people. This was a drama enterprise, involving taking puppet shows to schools in the region, with plays written specially for the purpose of enhancing children's awareness of stigma, disfigurement and disadvantage. One of their first productions was "There aren't many camels in Fife", a production asking questions about what constitutes normality and abnormality.

When hearing of the long journey which many make to the Centre in Fife, one is reminded of pilgrims travelling for example to Canterbury, and more recently to Lourdes, with the strong expectation of relief, and perhaps cure or regeneration. Visitors to Fife travel with hope, and with a predisposition to succeed. There may even be a tendency to see the possibility of positive outcome in proportion to the effort or discomfort sustained (as Festinger found in "When Prophecy Fails"[3]), rather than basing it on material facts.

The Disfigurement Guidance Centre also takes up individual situations, acting as advocate or champion for those who had had difficulty in obtaining a service, or have experienced prejudice or rejection. For example, early in 1989, they highlighted the story of a Welsh family who had been asked to remove their child from a playgroup; the child had a marked congenital facial blemish, and parents of the other children did not wish their children to play with him. The Disfigurement Guidance Centre raised public indignation about the family's experience, but they were also of practical help: they obtained the services of Ian Jackson (see Chapter Five) who agreed to operate on the child.

## Disadvantages of mutual help groups

The Trusts' experience of mutual support groups goes back to the early 1970s, when they set up such a group in Glasgow. What they found was that disfigured people found others' disfigurement more difficult to tolerate than their own, and it acted as a distorting mirror to their own appearance. The disfigured person was striving, chameleon-like, to be part of the crowd, an indistinguishable element of it. The group reduced this possibility, because the grouping together of people who had some feelings about being unattractive would detract from the overall need to re-integrate the person back into the full mainstream of society. The danger of the group lay in the maintenance of the separate enclosed setting which the patient had achieved as a temporary, necessary protection against public view and opinion. This is in direct contrast to the practice of Let's Face It groups to view hospitals as accepting, safe places.

The Trusts felt very strongly about the risks of putting people in a social setting where more powerful people could control less influential members. Such a process failed to recognise the unique skills of each individual, and the strengths which would ultimately lead to complete re- integration. By contrast, they believed that the professional could provide controlled guidance which in no way detracted from the self-motivation of the person.

The service provided by the Disfigurement Guidance Centre is a professional service. Doreen Trust is a teacher by training, and her husband an artist. They have achieved a high success rate with their individual advice and counselling sessions. They feel that this applies even more now than when they used to bring the service to others by travelling around the country. The commitment required to travel to Fife seems to have an overflow into the commitment to resume normal living. People who have travelled to the centre also talk about the value of having reflection time while travelling to and from Fife, while cut off from the distractions of daily living. This is viewed as a more positive approach than one which involves seeking the companionship of people with similar difficulties and image. In their view mutual help groups maximise the person's pre-occupation with the disfigurement, thereby slowing down the process of healing and re-integration. This is in direct conflict with the aims and practices of groups such as Let's Face It, and the value of the two approaches will be discussed below.

## Summary of characteristics of voluntary organisations concerned with disfigurement

The following chart draws together the themes described above, based on the responses of the groups when interviewed about their nature and purpose.

### Table 5.1
### Characteristics of Mutual Help Groups

| | Guinea Pig Club | Let's Face it | Disfigurement Guidance Centre |
|---|---|---|---|
| Originator | War-time RAF group | Woman patient with facial cancer | Teacher and artist husband |
| Whether disfigured | Yes | Yes | Yes |
| Aims:<br>- mutual support<br>- financial help<br>- counselling<br>- public awareness<br>- campaigning | Yes<br>Yes<br>Yes<br>No<br>No | Yes<br>No<br>Yes<br>Yes<br>Yes | Yes<br>No<br>Yes<br>Yes<br>Yes |
| Membership/association | Restricted | Open | Open |
| Conditions of membership | Burned or mutilated in World War II and treated at East Grinstead | Disfigurement or concern for interest | Disfigurement or concern or interest |
| Leadership | Elected | Charismatic | Self-selected |
| Advisory or management body | Yes | No (except in local group) | Yes |
| Activities | Reunions and individual welfare | Support groups, telephone and written contact | Counselling, advice, training |
| Local groups | No | Yes | No |
| Journal | Yes | Yes | Yes |
| Philanthropy or mutual aid | Mutual aid | Mutual aid | Philanthropy |

## Discussion

In the voluntary groups described in this chapter, the individual member participates with an expectation that the activity will be to his or her advantage, while also wishing to benefit the other members. The value in their eyes of having a group composed of people with similar needs to their own is the greater understanding which the members will have of the needs, strengths and weaknesses, and characteristics of each other. As one group leader told me, "No-one who is not facially disfigured can really understand what the problems are". Whether this is so remains to be seen, but what cannot be contested is that the members feel that it is true. For this reason mutual help groups exist in large numbers, frequently very specialist in their sphere of operation, often relating to one disease or disorder, or to a distinct social characteristic, such as single parenthood. But do they work - do they make the members feel better, improve their life, make it more tolerable, enhance their chances of resuming normal activities such as going to work, participating in relationships and family life? If the concept does work, why does it work - is the giving done with an expectation of immediate return, or is it a selfless act which does not require reciprocation, at least in the immediate?

The relationship between the members of a mutual help group for people with a disfigurement is not a commercial relationship, and it is not a professional one, even though some of its members stand in a professional position to some of the other members. It is principally one of giving and receiving, with no consideration for what might be gained from the giving, other than the right to receive in return when the need arises. Some members give more than others, according to their ability to do so, and some receive more, according to their need.

Titmuss would argue that there are many instances where the giver has no expectation of return, or where the likelihood of return is so remote that it does not influence the transaction either way. Blood donors have no immediate expectation of return, and indeed hope never to have cause to receive blood themselves. In this instance there exists what Wilensky and Lebeaux call "a degree of social distance between helped and helper".

> Social gifts and actions carrying no explicit or implicit right to a return gift or action are forms of 'creative altruism' (in Sorokin's words). They are creative in the sense that the self is realized with the help of anonymous others.... Manifestations of altruism in this sense may be thought of as self-love. But

they may also be thought of as giving life, or prolonging life or enriching life for anonymous others.[4]

This is echoed by Pinker, with reference to the residual model of welfare:

.... the distinctive feature of good citizenship is the exchange relationship based on reciprocity and bilateral transfers.[5]

He goes on to say that the exchange is motivated by economic forces, and that in this context citizens "are acting out of self-interest - enlightened though it may be - rather than altruism". This is true of the mutual help group, in which there is some expectation or contract, however informal, which influences the behaviour of the members. They agree to exchange things of value, such as sympathy, understanding, advice and support, and the more they participate, the stronger their belief in the power and ability of themselves as group members. People who enter into an exchange relationship, if they are rewarded, will be motivated to participate in further exchanges, as they view each other in favourable terms. One kind of action has been rewarded - so they are pre-disposed to reward others.

The fact that the two men have now rewarded one another ... may lead them to revise the original exchange so as to make it more rewarding to them both. The stimulus each presents to the other has become to some degree more favourable. Accordingly each may begin to direct new actions towards the other on the presumption that these will be rewarded too.[6]

While the transaction within a mutual help group may not be so explicit, there is likely to be an element of such calculation within any individual's decision to participate. Not everyone can or should develop such a balance in their relationships, and some can tolerate much more ambiguity than this model would suggest.

## The role of the professional in the voluntary group

The participant professionals are drawing together voluntary and statutory effort, which, according to Pinker, is required because of the size and complexity of contemporary social issues and problems. Voluntary groups are needed, and professional effort is also required;

it would be sad and unproductive if these two forces were not in some way in harmony with each other:

It is morally right for civic involvement in welfare policy to go beyond the traditional boundaries and forms of self-help.[7]

The professional group leaders appear to be giving more than receiving, if the calculation is made on the basis of the extent of support given and received. They would say, however, that they receive as much or more by their act of giving than their members receive, because of the satisfaction which the altruistic gift offers.

The professionals who act as group leaders or convenors have not experienced facial disfigurement for themselves. This must be considered alongside the strongly held belief amongst disfigured people that no one can understand their needs who has not suffered as they have. It is the common suffering which is the key to the whole idea of mutual support - "Stick together and no power on earth can break you". The professionals who participate (and often lead) are seen as a vital link between the disfigured person and key people on whom he or she is dependent, such as surgeons and radiotherapists. This is particularly important when the individual person feels that there is lack of understanding on the part of those senior professionals - a situation often referred to by Christine Piff. It does, however, detract from the original suggestion that no one but the disfigured person can understand - the professional is seen as mediator between those who do not understand and the person who is disfigured.


## Do mutual help groups work?

To this day, the objectives of the Guinea Pig Club continue to be met. Is this through mutuality, or the benevolence of individuals or organisations? Certainly the welfare element of the club's activities is underwritten by the R.A.F. Benevolent Fund. The club does not meet all its own needs, particularly financial. Clinical needs too are met by professionals. However, the personal support and encouragement which many of the members need and do receive is provided predominantly by members themselves. In particular it is provided by designated members who are felt to be in the strongest position to do so, and are nominated as officers of the club for this purpose. This is not a fully reciprocal arrangement, inasmuch as some members will never have given, and others will never have received. In straight exchange terms a transaction has not taken place with the intention of replicating it in reciprocal form at a future date. However, because of the bonds which exist between all members, there is trust enough to make it work. The givers believe in what they're giving, and those who receive do not mind receiving unilaterally; they trust those who are helping them because of their common experience. They also all know that if the tables were turned - if the dependent became strong and the helpers became dependent - the arrangement would be just as successful. There is therefore potential for reciprocity even if this is never fully actualised.

The Guinea Pig Club arose from very special circumstances, the severe mutilation and burning of air force personnel on active service, and the pioneering days of reconstructive surgery. Although war and injury are not unique to that point in history, the exact circumstances which gave rise to and sustained the club are unlikely to be repeated. The issues of comradeship and heroism were at least as important as injury and reconstruction, and so the Guinea Pigs form a special group of their own which we hope will never need to be replicated.

A contemporary parallel exists in the case of Simon Weston, a Welsh Guardsman who was burned severely in the course of the Falklands conflict. After years of reconstruction and rehabilitation, Weston has now established Weston Spirit, which enables young people to develop initiative and self-reliance. His was an individualistic response - making positive use of the reputation which he acquired through the three B.B.C. documentaries about him, he established contact with all groups and individuals needed to enable him to be successful in his trust. Participation in a group of people in similar circumstances to himself would not have had the same result.

Doreen and Peter Trust say that mutual help groups do not work; not only that, but they slow down the process of the individual making a full come-back into society, by reinforcing the acceptability of the disfigurement, or by overwhelming the individual with the appearance of other members of the group. Yet literally thousands of people, here and in other countries, find them a comfort and a strength, saying literally the opposite of what the Trusts say, that the group helps them to feel normal and acceptable again:

> [they] have an immense normalising effect on members.... [they] seem to go past the pathology to recognise and nurture members' strengths and competence.[8]

Here we have a strong disagreement: many say that groups help make them feel normal; others say that normality cannot be reinforced or restored by a group with such evident differences from the normal. Whether groups can be described as having a normalising effect must be challenged, as the group itself is not a normal experience. Wolfensberger's definition of normalisation is:

> Utilisation of means which are as culturally normative as possible, in order to establish and/or maintain personal behaviours and characteristics which are as culturally normative as possible.[9]

Normalisation is therefore a process and a goal; mutual help groups match the goal, but not the process. The much simpler earlier Scandinavian definition of normalisation does have more tolerance of processes or means which are not necessarily normative. In the context of people with mental handicaps, normalisation is described as:

> Letting the mentally retarded obtain an existence as close to the normal as possible.[10]

By either definition, groups which look inward to the members do not provide a normal experience; it is the fact that members see each other as special which gives them strength. They should therefore not be seen as normalising.

Not everyone likes groups, and not everyone takes comfort from seeing those in like circumstances. The Trusts' forthright approach is of value to such people, and there are many illustrations in their files which prove this. However, theirs is a service model, provided by professionals, and not everyone is prepared to come to professionals, when they feel that, rightly or wrongly, professionals have contributed to their feelings of isolation and low worth. For this reason mutual help groups, which for once leave the control with the disfigured person, have a value:

> They offer very real relief from isolation and fear, in ways that even the most sympathetic doctor cannot approach.[11]

This is the view of an American physician (Gaioni,K. New Physician, 1988), who frequently "prescribes" self-help groups for her patients. It reinforces the views of the leaders of such groups, and of the members, who by their very participation are acknowledging the value of the experience. There may come a point, however, when participation becomes unproductive. The Trusts would argue that the group member may stick at a certain point of the rehabilitative process, unable to proceed because the other members are reinforcing the advantages of membership. For example, the very exclusivity of the Guinea Pig Club, which aims to give the members a positive image of themselves, might encourage members to stay within these exclusive boundaries, and not move forward. Meanwhile, for many the groups offer comfort and companionship, and a feeling of worth which otherwise would be difficult to attain

> Self-help groups provide patients with the rare opportunity to learn from positive role models - those who have been there. They often experience an increased sense of needed self-worth and self-esteem as they begin to see how their experience with adversity enables them to help others in the mutual aid group.[12]

For those with a facial disfigurement, the world may seem a very unaccepting place. While influencing public attitudes and responses is a crucial objective, this must not be at the expense of the feelings of the present generation of disfigured people, who need to have their own worth enhanced while the long job of public education continues. They must seek whatever means of survival and improvement they have at their disposal, and maintain positive attitudes about themselves and each other. In the long run, does it matter whether the process of group membership is culturally normative or not, as long members achieve satisfaction and fulfilment from participation? Some people are gregarious and gain a lot from group activity; others feel that groups reinforce their own self-doubts and low self-rating. Facially disfigured people will make their choice about which support model they gain most by using.

The fact that so many members join mutual help groups such as Let's Face It suggests that there is a need to be met; does the group meet that need? Only the disfigured person can answer this. The enthusiasm with which the network is greeted and sustained is a large part of the answer. Disfigured people continually make the point that they have a unique or special feature, and no one understands them who does not share that special attribute:

> What came out of that meeting was the clear need that there should be support groups all over the country for us to be able to meet with each other and to share our upsets (and our joys).For when it comes to the crunch no matter how lovely

162

other people are to us, it is only when we meet others like ourselves that we get that real understanding. That understanding is not borne out of theory or pity, but out of experience of the same or similar situation.[13]

This need for understanding is widely expressed, not by the founder alone but also by members of the network, such as the woman quoted immediately above. The need is there, and the group members say that Let's Face It satisfies the need. In the same way that one does not rate the value of other friends in functional terms, so it is impossible to rate the performance of the members of Let's Face It, or for that matter of its founder. Its objectives are described to a large extent in terms of the characteristics of friendship - "That's what the Network is all about, caring and sharing." Whether the physical and social functioning of its members is enhanced, or whether their psychological functioning is measurably better, is not demonstrable within this framework; indeed members would shrink from expressing the outcome of their activities in those terms. They want to be friends, special friends, with people who have experienced the same strong feelings about disfigurement as they have.

We are special people. There are a lot of us, but we form a minority in society at large. We are coming together in the Network for mutual support, to help each other to face it.[14]

Quite simply, friends are getting together to help each other to face it. They say they do, and no one can contradict them, as 'facing it' is such a personal matter. It might be argued that a group of people with like problems getting together serves only to exacerbate those problems. They literally act as mirrors to each other, reminding each other of their morbidity. It can be said (and this will be discussed in detail later) that this is particularly so of people with a very visible disorder such as a facial disfigurement. As with many other special groups, it has to be admitted that it works with some and not with others. The coming together and supporting each other which takes place in Let's Face It is reminiscent of the "sticking together" of the Guinea Pigs. It would be understandable if individuals felt it reminded them of what they might have looked like or indeed what they may look like in the future if malignancy recurs, but many do find it a positive asset - for them voluntary groups do work.

163

## Notes

1. Piff, C., 1985 *Let's Face It*, Victor Gollancz, London.
2. Salmon, J. 1987 'Special People', *Let's Face It Newsletter*, April.
3. Festinger, L. et al., 1964, *When Prophecy Fails*, Harper and Row, London.
4. Titmuss, R.M., 1973 *The Gift Relationship*, Penguin, Harmondsworth.
5. Pinker, R., 1979 *The Idea of Welfare*, Heinemann, London, p. 6.
6. Homans, G.C., 1974 *Social Behaviour, Its Elementary Forms*, Harcourt Brace Jovanovich, New York.
7. Pinker, R., op. cit., p. 5.
8. Gaioni, K., 1988, 'Rx: Self-Help,' *The New Physician*, July-August, p. 33.
9. Wolfensberger, W., 1972, *The Principle of Normalisation in Human Services*, National Institute on Mental Retardation, Toronto. p. 28.
10. op. cit., p. 27.
11. Gaioni, op. cit.
12. ibid.
13. Salmon, op. cit.
14. ibid.

# PART III
# AN EMPIRICAL
# ENQUIRY

# 6 Methodology

The broad aim of the study was to understand the characteristics and needs of those who have undergone facial surgery, thereby to cast light on the broader characteristics and needs of others who are facially disfigured.

There were two more specific objectives in mind, as follows:

1. To test the hypotheses which emerged from the review of the literature. These are listed below;

2. To assist in focusing the efforts of helping professions, particularly social work, by providing a framework for assisting those who are facially disfigured.

**The hypotheses**

From the material reviewed in Parts I and II, there emerged the following hypotheses:

1. Facially disfigured people are stigmatised. It is therefore expected that people will deal differently with those who have undergone facial surgery;

2. The patients in the study will seek ways of managing their differentness. Of the strategies suggested by Goffman, covering, withdrawing and fighting are the most likely;

3. The patients are likely to retain acceptance by those close to them, and the greatest tension will be felt when

meeting strangers;

4.     The patients will feel separated from others by virtue of difficulties with speech and eating, and by their appearance;

5.     Good communication between surgeon and patient enables trust to develop. This in turn affects the patient's acceptance of surgery;

6.     Social workers play a major part in the rehabilitation process;

7.     Patients who are accepting of surgery and changed appearance will have a distinctive social profile;

8.     Patients with facial cancer will tend to be of lower social classes, more male than female, in late middle age, and with a tendency to smoke and drink heavily;

9.     Surgery which has to be performed because of head and neck cancer will tend to be accompanied by signs of depression, dissatisfaction with the body, reduction in quality of life, and family tensions;

10.     Those who function better after illness and treatment will be those with strong and intact egos, older people with a settled way of life, and those with a good family support network;

11.     Early detection of head and neck cancer will increase the chances of survival;

12.     Patients will benefit from the combined efforts of a range of professionals more than from those same professionals operating independently from each other;

13.     Patients are assisted in their recovery by keeping control of their treatment and management;

14.     People will vary in the amount of reconstructive work which they feel they need, for own self-respect, and to

make them presentable to others;

15.     Facial disfigurement through surgery will cause a major upheaval in people's lives;

16.     Patients who have had facial surgery are likely to experience feelings characteristic of bereavement, since changed facial appearance is a form of loss.


## The sample

Obtaining the sample was difficult; at the beginning of the study, I was working as a principal social worker in a teaching hospital, the Royal Victoria Infirmary in Newcastle upon Tyne, but I was not working directly in the plastic surgery or oral surgery departments. It was therefore necessary to negotiate access with the plastic surgeons in the hospital. After much discussion, the surgeons agreed to assist, but problems arose when defining the type of patient whom they would refer. Broadly, there were three categories of patient who could be considered:

1.     Those with facial cancer;

2.     Those who had sustained a physical trauma, such as a road accident or a burn;

3.     Those who had been disfigured from birth, and were now choosing to undergo corrective surgery.

Those with congenital deformities were first considered, but it was not possible to gain access to them. The surgeons were concerned that the introduction of a research element into the association between the surgeon and those with congenital deformities might jeopardise the distinctive relationship which tends to exist between surgeon and patient. The patient, whether child or adult, frequently needs encouragement or reassurance when deciding whether to proceed, and on occasions even more so when deciding to continue treatment. The surgeon sees himself or herself as having a very special counselling role, which can be taken by no one else, since a high degree of trust needs to be developed between the patient and the person who is going to alter his or her face. The surgeons did not wish to upset this relationship by the introduction of another person, whose focus would necessarily be those areas which were being discussed by surgeon and patient, and so they chose not to refer for the study patients who had a congenital deformity.

Trauma patients were unpredictable, both in absolute numbers, and in when they were going to present. They were a small number of highly disfigured and injured people, who were very much worthy of study; however, given the outsider status of the researcher, it was not possible to organise access systematically and over a reasonable period of time.

Treatment of facial cancer patients was more regular. A joint clinic was held every fortnight at the radiotherapy department at Newcastle General Hospital, between the plastic surgeons, the radiotherapists and the oral physicians. This clinic considered new patients, decided on the best means of treatment, and reviewed patients after surgery. In effect, they reviewed patients on a permanent basis in case of recurrence of cancer. It was therefore agreed that the surgeons would refer for the research any patients who had recently undergone surgery for facial cancer. For other patients the agreed treatment was radiotherapy of one kind or another, and these patients were not included; for people with facial cancer, the principal disfiguring component is the treatment - the surgery itself, and in the case of those treated by radiotherapy, this is not so.

A further qualifier was made to the sample; not all head and neck cancer patients have evident tumours on the outside tissue of their face; many present with intra-oral tumours. These were included in the study, since they were part of the same group of tumours histologically, and since their treatment tended to involve cutting open the external tissue of the face, usually leaving a scar, however minimal. In addition, the study showed that felt disfigurement was not necessarily related to the extent of external mutilation, and damage such as a partially removed tongue was just as disabling and mutilating as a more visible excision.

A protocol was agreed that as soon as the patient returned to the clinic for follow-up after surgery, the surgeon would seek his or her consent to participation in the study. If consent was obtained, the surgeon would send to the researcher a completed note of referral; these notes were drafted by the researcher, and left in the clinic in plentiful supplies. Generally, therefore, it would be possible to interview the patients for the study around six weeks after surgery had taken place.

A total sample number of 100 patients was agreed on. It was felt that this would provide a sufficient range of patients for the purposes of describing the needs and characteristics of patients, and of determining what social needs should be met by a social work service. It was expected that the assembling of these 100 people might take up to one year. The process began early in 1986. In fact, in the early months of 1986, no referrals were forthcoming, and this was giving the researcher great cause for concern. Alternative sources of referrals were considered, and two chance encounters widened the options substantially.

The first was with a friend, who had contacts with the oral and maxillo-facial surgery department at Sunderland General Hospital. The two oral surgeons there expressed great interest in the study, and offered to participate. From conversation with them it emerged that oral and facial cancer is treated by a range of clinicians, and surgical treatment is handled either by plastic surgeons or by oral surgeons. Which discipline offers treatment is largely determined by the original G.P. or dental referral. The study will show that dental surgeons play a significant role in the detection of head and neck cancer, and they would be pre-disposed to refer such patients to oral surgeons, who have very strong associations with dental surgeons (oral surgeons are trained in medicine, surgery and dentistry).

At this point a significant variation was considered in the protocol for collecting patients for the sample. The Sunderland surgeons invited the research staff to their regular Monday morning clinic, to meet patients for themselves, and to invite their participation in the study. This offer was accepted immediately, and several patients were enlisted on the first day. Thereafter it became evident that personal attendance by the research staff at the clinic was the only sure way of recruiting patients. Sunderland General Hospital was the greatest provider of patients throughout the study.

The second contact was with a plastic surgeon in Leeds, who expressed interest in the study, and invited me to observe a facial reconstruction operation at St. James' Hospital, Leeds. This experience has already been described in the introduction. Thereafter, the same patient agreed to participate in the study, as did one further patient from Leeds.

With the knowledge and experience that personal contact was important, the Newcastle plastic surgeons were once more approached. They apologised for their failure to refer, and agreed that the researcher should attend their fortnightly joint head and neck cancer clinic. From this several more patients were obtained.

By this time, late 1987, it was evident that the net needed to be

171

widened even further if anything approaching the full 100 patient sample was going to be found. The advice of the Sunderland oral surgeons was sought, and they helped in two ways. The first was an introduction to the joint clinic which they held with oral surgeons from Teesside, at which they discussed treatment and sometimes took decisions to carry out joint surgery. I began to attend these joint clinics on the same basis as my attendance at Newcastle and Sunderland, and a substantial number of patients was found who agreed to participate. The second suggestion was to contact a range of oral surgeons in the north of England and in Scotland, all known personally to the Sunderland surgeons, asking them to participate. This was a big step, partly because it would involve much travelling, and partly because the involvement of further treatment centres was adding further dimensions to the characteristics of the patients.

In the event, three centres agreed to help. One, in Liverpool, subsequently withdrew, and a further Liverpool hospital produced only one patient. An oral surgeon from Airdrie in Strathclyde was happy to be involved, and a further four patients were found from that source.

In all, by the end of 1988, a total of 71 patients was found, and it was decided that a halt should be called; otherwise the work would not be completed within a reasonable timescale.


**The research interviews**

Two interviews were carried out with each of the 71 people in the sample. The patients were identified in the clinic, often before surgery, but they were not asked for their help until they attended the follow-up clinic after surgery, and it was seen that they were sufficiently recovered to engage in discussion.

The first interview took place as soon as possible after surgery. This tended to be around six to eight weeks after the operation, by which time the individuals were home, recovering from the immediate physical impact of the surgery, but still able to remember vividly the feelings and events leading up to treatment, and the treatment itself. It was felt important to ensure that they were seen at this point, since they would be unlikely to recall such details to the same extent if a longer period had elapsed.

The second interview took place one year after the first. It was hoped and expected that by this time the patients and their families would have begun to resume their normal lives, or would have adjusted to whatever differences and constraints the illness and treatment had imposed. It was hoped that insights would be obtained into the stresses and difficulties encountered, and the ways in which these were faced and resolved by patients and their families. On the other hand, if they had not been resolved, it was important to understand what were the lasting effects of illness and mutilating surgery.

Of the 71 original patients, only 53 survived until the time of second interview. Of those 53, one preferred not to be interviewed, and so the second interviews relate to a much smaller sample. However, the fact that 18 people did not survive gave the opportunity to consider their characteristics, and to consider whether they contained any special features which contrasted with those who did survive.

**Interview schedules**

Two distinct interview formats were used, one for the early interview and one for the follow-up session. In content the two were similar to each other, so that comparative and contrasting information could be obtained.

For the first interview, a pilot version was used for the first ten patients, but only minor amendments were made as a result, and so all of these ten patients were used in the main study. The experience of using the first year schedule influenced the design of the second, and lessons learned were applied in its format as well as content. Most of these were about the order of questions, and the design of a format which lent itself more easily to analysis. However, some developments related more to content, such as the inclusion in the second schedule of questions relating to alcohol consumption, which emerged as an issue which it would have been useful to cover from the beginning. Copies of each schedule are given in Appendix I.

The schedules are made up of a combination of coded and open questions. The closed or coded answers were analysed with computer assistance, using SPSSX. The content of the open, more narrative, answers, was also analysed, and used to amplify, illustrate and qualify the coded responses.

The following areas were covered by the interviews:

1       Social profile of the patient;

2.       Becoming ill and receiving treatment;

3.       Impact on job and finance;

4.       Impact on social life;

5.       Facial appearance.


## Carrying out the interviews

The interviews were conducted by a total of five interviewers, all of them qualified and experienced social workers. The use of social workers to interview was a deliberate choice, first so that a social, and non-clinical perspective would be the prevailing one in the results, and second so that the circumstances and feelings of people in a vulnerable situation would be acknowledged and where necessary responded to. Where a need was felt for further help, the interviewer discussed it with the patient, and came to agreement about referral on - to the surgeon, the local authority social worker, or to the general practitioner.

I carried out a number of interviews myself at each of the two stages, to ensure that the schedules were robust enough, and in order to be as sensitive as possible to the situations of the interviewees.

All of the interviewers were briefed in detail by me, and all carried out the interviews in a similar manner. The schedule was not completed in front of the patient, but the interviewers had with them a checklist of prompts to ensure that all the required areas were covered. Where they felt it necessary, they also jotted down notes, with the agreement of the interviewees. Immediately after the interviews, and always within twenty-four hours, the schedules were completed. Where additional important material emerged, which could not be accommodated within the framework of the schedule, the interviewers wrote additional notes, which have proved invaluable in assisting with the analysis. These referred in part to the manner in which the individual interviews were conducted (for example when a spouse was trying to answer for the patient and not letting him or her speak for himself or herself), and in part to additional insights into the circumstances of the individual.

The interviews with all 71 patients who agreed to take part were recorded in this way, and analysed. Their responses are described and analysed in the following chapter.

# 7 The experience of illness and treatment

**Profile of patients**

There were 71 patients in the sample. Table 7.1 describes the gender distribution, which is almost exactly a 2:1 ratio of male to female.

**Table 7.1**
**Gender of Patients    N = 71**

|        |     | %     |
|--------|-----|-------|
| Male   | 47  | 66.2  |
| Female | 24  | 33.8  |
| Total  | 71  | 100.0 |

The ages of the patients, summarised in Table 7.2, ranged from 35 years to 94 years. Both of these extreme cases were men. In general, however, the men were closer to their mean age than the women.

**Table 7.2**
**Age of Patients    N = 71**

|          | Male | Female | Total |
|----------|------|--------|-------|
| Mean age | 61   | 65     | 62    |
| S.D.     | 13   | 15     | 13    |
| Min.     | 35   | 39     | 35    |
| Max      | 94   | 85     | 94    |

Table 7.3 provides further detail of the age distribution; U.K. comparisons for each age group are also given. These were 1989 figures.

**Table 7.3**
**Age Distribution of Patients     N = 71**
(column percentages in brackets)

|  |  |  | U.K. |
|---|---|---|---|
| 30 < 40 | 5 | (7.0) | (23.3) |
| 40 < 50 | 8 | (11.3) | (22.2) |
| 50 < 60 | 15 | (21.1) | (18.8) |
| 60 < 70 | 19 | (26.8) | (17.6) |
| 70 < 80 | 18 | (25.4) | (11.8) |
| 80+ | 6 | (8.5) | (6.3) |
| Total | 71 | (100.0) | (100.0) |

Seventy-three per cent of the patients were within the age range from 50 to 80 years.

Where possible an appraisal of social class was made, using the Registrar-General's classification. Where this was impossible or inappropriate because the patient had never worked or had not done so for a very long time, he or she was simply described as "unclassified." Retired people have been classified according to their previous occupation; "unclassified" relates particularly to those who had never worked. Although 21 per cent fell into this group, it could be observed that most of them lived in relatively modest or poor circumstances. In later analyses they will be treated as manual. Social class is described in Table 7.4.

**Table 7.4**
**Social Class     N = 71**
(column percentages in brackets)

|  | Male | Female | Total |
|---|---|---|---|
| Professional | 4 (8.5) | 1 (4.2) | 5 (7.0) |
| Intermediate | 1 (2.1) | nil | 1 (1.4) |
| Skilled non-manual | 2 (4.3) | 2 (8.3) | 4 (5.6) |

'continued'

| | | | |
|---|---|---|---|
| Skilled manual | 9 (19.1) | 1 (4.2) | 10 (14.1) |
| Partly-skilled man | 22 (46.8) | 2 (8.3) | 24 (33.8) |
| Unskilled | 9 (19.1) | 3 (12.5) | 12 (16.9) |
| Unclassified | nil | 15 (62.5) | 15 (21.1) |
| | | | |
| Total | 47(100.0) | 24(100.0) | 71(100.0) |

This was a group of people of predominantly manual occupation - 14 per cent non-manual and 86 per cent manual.

No men were unclassified; they had all at some stage been at work or classified in terms of work. Thus, all the 15 patients who were described as "unclassified" were women, and this represented the largest group of women, 62 per cent.

To summarise the profile of the whole group, it can be said that most of the patients are in the fifty to eighty years age range, and are or have been engaged in manual occupations (or cannot be classified). The next two tables provide a similar analysis for male and female patients separately. Table 7.5 considers the social class and age of the male patients.

### Table 7.5
### Social Class by Age - Male Patients    N = 47

| | Age | | | | | | |
|---|---|---|---|---|---|---|---|
| | 30<40 | 41<50 | 51<60 | 61<70 | 71<80 | 80+ | Total |
| Professional | 1 | nil | nil | 1 | 1 | 1 | 4 |
| Intermediate | nil | nil | nil | 1 | nil | nil | 1 |
| Skilled non-manual | nil | nil | nil | 1 | 1 | nil | 2 |
| Skilled manual | 1 | nil | 3 | 1 | 3 | 1 | 9 |
| Part-skilled man. | nil | 4 | 6 | 8 | 3 | 1 | 22 |
| Unskilled manual | 1 | 2 | 2 | 2 | 2 | nil | 9 |
| Unclassified | nil | nil | nil | nil | nil | nil | |
| | | | | | | | |
| Total | 3 | 6 | 11 | 14 | 10 | 3 | 47 |

It will be noted that there are few young non-manual patients - only one under the age of sixty. There are no men who have not been classified according to occupation. The largest single group, 29%, are partly-skilled men aged 50 to 70. It is the men who contribute most to the picture of ageing manual workers. Table 7.6 offers the same analysis for women.

### Table 7.6
### Social Class by Age - Female Patients    N = 24

|  | Age | | | | | | |
| --- | --- | --- | --- | --- | --- | --- | --- |
|  | 30<40 | 41<50 | 51<60 | 61<70 | 71<80 | 80+ | Total |
| Professional | 1 | nil | nil | nil | nil | nil | 1 |
| Intermediate | nil | nil | nil | nil | nil | nil | nil |
| Skilled non-manual | nil | 1 | nil | nil | 1 | nil | 2 |
| Skilled manual | nil | nil | nil | nil | 1 | nil | 1 |
| Part-skilled man. | nil | nil | 1 | nil | 1 | nil | 2 |
| Unskilled manual | nil | nil | nil | 2 | 1 | nil | 3 |
| Unclassified | 1 | 1 | 3 | 1 | 6 | 3 | 15 |
| Total | 2 | 2 | 4 | 3 | 10 | 3 | 24 |

The majority of women have had no paid employment throughout their lives, and so could not be classified. The biggest single group of women was those six women in their seventies (25%) who had never had paid employment. The majority were therefore unclassified - 62.3%, and the largest single group were in their seventies - 42%.

## Household composition

Slightly over one quarter of those interviewed, 29.6%, lived alone, and most of the rest lived with a spouse. Composition of household at the time of first interview is described in Table 7.7.

### Table 7.7
### Members of Household    N = 71
(more than one response is possible)

|  | Male | Female | Total |
| --- | --- | --- | --- |
| Lives alone | 7 | 14 | 21 |

'continued'

| | | | |
|---|---|---|---|
| With spouse/equiv | 34 | 9 | 43 |
| With parent/s | 3 | 0 | 3 |
| With child/ren | 1 | 1 | 2 |
| With other relative | 2 | 0 | 2 |
| With non-relative | 1 | 0 | 1 |

More than half of the women (58%) lived alone, and almost all of the remainder lived with a spouse. For men by far the largest proportion (72%) lived with a spouse. Few of either gender lived with a household member other than a spouse - three (all men) lived with their parents, two had children living with them, two lived with another relative, and one lived with a non-relative.

29.6% of the sample lived alone. This is higher than the U.K. figures for single households. In 1987, for example, 25% of all households were households of single people.

## Summary of profile of interviewees

Two thirds of the 71 patients were male, and one third were female. They ranged in age from 35 years to 94, with a mean of 62. More than two thirds were (or had been) manual workers, and most of the one fifth who could not be classified lived in relatively modest or poor circumstances. The largest group within the patients was of working class men over 50, most of whom had already ceased to work before becoming ill.

More women than men in the sample lived alone - 14 compared to 7, and in proportional terms this represents 58.3 per cent of the women and 14.8 per cent of the men.

## Becoming ill and undergoing treatment

The period during which the clinical condition had existed before surgery was undertaken varied from patient to patient. Clear trends are slightly blurred by the fact that for a small number of patients this was not their first occurrence of cancer or their first episode of treatment, but rather a stage in a longer process. There are two distinct groups: new patients and returning patients. This helps to explain why, for

179

example, for eight patients there was a gap of more than a year between the discovery of the condition and this current phase of treatment. What is reported here, in Table 7.8, is the patient's own perception and memory of events.

### Table 7.8
### Time Before Treatment that Patient was Aware that Condition
### Existed  N = 71
(column percentages in brackets)

|  | Male | Female | Total |
|---|---|---|---|
| < 1 week | 3 (10.7) | nil | 3 (4.2) |
| 1 < 4 weeks | 13 (27.7) | 5 (20.9) | 18 (25.3) |
| 5 < 8 weeks | 9 (19.2) | 3 (12.5) | 12 (16.8) |
| 8 weeks < 6 mths | 13 (27.7) | 7 (29.2) | 20 (28.0) |
| 6 months < 1 year | 6 (12.7) | 4 (66.7) | 10 (14.0) |
| 1 year + | 3 (6.4) | 5 (20.8) | 8 (11.3) |
| Total | 47(100.0) | 24(100.0) | 71(100.0) |

For a small number of patients the response and treatment had been almost immediate (4.2 per cent). Just over a quarter had been aware of the condition for less than four weeks before surgery. As mentioned above, eight patients (11.3 per cent) had had the condition for more than a year - one patient had been under treatment for about ten years, and this episode was just one part of a long reconstructive process.

Generally, women had been aware of having a problem for longer than men. For 67 per cent of women the condition had existed for two months or more before treatment, compared with 47 per cent of men.

Table 7.9 describes the responses to the question : "Who identified the fact that you had a problem?"

### Table 7.9
### Who Identified the Problem?  N = 71
(column percentages in brackets)

|  | Male | Female | Total |
|---|---|---|---|
| Self | 25 (53.2) | 11 (45.8) | 36 (50.7) |

'continued'

| | | | |
|---|---|---|---|
| Spouse | 2 (4.3) | 2 (8.3) | 4 (5.6) |
| G.P. | 7 (14.9) | 3 (12.5) | 10 (14.1) |
| Consultant | 2 (4.3) | nil | 2 (2.8) |
| Dentist | 10 (21.3) | 6 (25.0) | 16 (22.5) |
| Other | 1 (2.1) | 2 (8.3) | 3 (4.2) |

Half of the patients had acknowledged a serious problem themselves before seeking attention. For a few, the spouse had raised concern. The other key groups for highlighting the problem were dentist and G.P., so that virtually all were aware by the time they got to the consultant that something serious was the matter. The dentist was a most significant person in the discovery of malignancy - in more than one fifth of the cases. There are some slight gender differences - the dentist played slightly more of a part in identifying the problem for women than for men, and slightly more men than women identified for themselves that they had a problem.

### The stay in hospital

Most people spent from one to three weeks in hospital, although the extended stays of a few people meant that the mean was around four weeks. In relation to contemporary surgical practice, these are long episodes.

**Table 7.10**
**Length of Stay in Hospital    N = 71**
(column percentages in brackets)

| | Male | Female | Total |
|---|---|---|---|
| < 1 week | 9 (19.1) | 4 (16.7) | 13 (18.3) |
| 1 < 2 weeks | 13 (27.7) | 7 (29.2) | 20 (28.2) |
| 2 < 3 weeks | 9 (19.1) | 9 (37.5) | 18 (23.4) |
| 3 < 8 weeks | 9 (19.1) | 3 (12.6) | 12 (16.8) |
| 9 <26 weeks | 7 (14.9) | 1 (4.2) | 8 (11.2) |
| Total | 47(100.0) | 24(100.0) | 71(100.0) |

Around 46 per cent of both men and women go home from hospital in less than two weeks. However, while most of the remaining women (37%) go home within three weeks, more men stay longer, 19 per cent up to two months, and 15 per cent up to six months - hence the mean of four weeks.

Patients were asked to comment on their experience by describing who had been of help to them while in hospital, and in what ways. The responses are summarised in Table 7.11.

**Table 7.11**
**Help Given by Professionals and Others    N = 71**
(more than one response is possible)

Resource - information, listening, counselling, finding advice

| | | | | |
|---|---|---|---|---|
| Surgeon | 4 | 32 | 13 | 4 |
| Psychiatrist | nil | nil | 1 | nil |
| G.P. | 4 | 6 | 3 | 1 |
| Priest etc. | nil | nil | 4 | nil |
| Social worker | nil | nil | 4 | nil |
| Relative/friend | nil | 1 | 17 | nil |
| Nurse | 1 | 11 | 20 | nil |
| Other | nil | 1 | 2 | nil |

Patients described the professionals and others who had been helpful, and the ways in which they had been useful. In addition to the specific responses given in the table, 18 said that everyone had been generally helpful, and did not wish to single out individuals.

Throughout the interviews there was little criticism of hospital services. Surgeons were mentioned frequently as helpful people, in a range of situations. Their primary function of clinical treatment was not the issue here - that was not discussed directly. They were seen by four people as resource brokers, and by 32 as providing information or advice, about outcome, prognosis, and other issues such as the management of a dressing or a prosthesis. They were also seen by 13 respondents as people who would just listen to the patient and relatives, and in four instances they were seen to offer a more serious counselling service.

General practitioners provided help to a significant number of people, but they were not seen to provide as much of a listening ear as do the surgeons; one might have expected the traditional role of family doctor to have contained more of this element. There was a small number of people who felt disappointed or bitter because a G.P. had failed to diagnose the condition earlier.

The traditional role of the priest or minister might have been expected to include listening in times of trouble, but only four people mentioned the minister's help (all in this listening role).

Only four mentioned that the social worker had performed such a service. The fact that social work occupies so small a place in the work of helping individuals over such a difficult process is of great concern in the context of this study, as the need to enhance social work's contribution to this field was one of the reasons why the study was undertaken in the first place.

Nursing staff provided the greatest "listening" support, and they were also seen as providers of information or advice.

Friends and relatives were also seen as significant, chiefly in the "listening" role.

Some felt that the imparting of the diagnosis could have been handled more sensitively, and many felt that further explicit support could have been offered. The need for such support was overwhelmingly stressed by patients. Table 7.12 describes when patients felt help was most needed.

### Table 7.12
### When Help was Needed    N = 71
(More than one response is possible)

| | | |
|---|---|---|
| At diagnosis | 43 | (60.6) |
| Before surgery | 41 | (57.7) |
| After surgery | 63 | (88.7) |

More than half felt that help should be available at all times, but the clearest message of all is that 89% felt that after the operation help and support should be available. For some it was indeed available, but the general experience was that after the major treatment had been carried out, much of the support faded out. It would appear that patients would like in some way to maintain contact with the treatment centre, in addition to the clinical follow-up appointments. When faced with the task of beginning the rest of their lives, once the acute phase is over, isolation and disadvantage is most felt.

## Outcome of surgery

At the time of first interview, 70 per cent of the patients said that the surgery had been successful. This included some who still said that further surgery was intended. The surgery was successful in the sense of eradicating malignancy. In most instances the reconstruction of the face was seen to be a separate, additional and less invasive task. Ten per cent said that treatment had not been successful, and one fifth were not sure whether the treatment had been successful or not; this seems a realistic judgement on outcome.

At the time of the first interviews (which were conducted within a short time after surgery), only a quarter of the patients felt better than previously (i.e. before surgery). A third felt about the same as previously, and 42 per cent said that they felt worse, with symptoms including continued pain, nausea (some patients then went on to receive radiotherapy), loss of appetite, functional difficulties (speech and eating) and general feeling of being unwell.

## Smoking

Oral surgeons stress to their patients the advisability of giving up smoking. Smoking has been found to be strongly associated with head and neck cancer. For this reason, patients were asked about their smoking habits. The responses are summarised in Table 7.13.

**Table 7.13**
**Smoking    N = 71**

|                          |    |   %  |
|--------------------------|----|------|
| Smokes                   | 28 | 39.4 |
| Recently gave up smoking | 9  | 12.7 |
| Gave up long ago         | 6  | 8.5  |
| Has never smoked         | 28 | 39.4 |

Almost 40 per cent of the group is still smoking, and only 13 per cent have given up recently, usually in association with the onset of illness. Looking at the recent smokers, 37, three quarters, are still smoking.

Several patients commented that they were aware of the risks, but preferred not to give up. At least one person interviewed had acquired a further primary lesion - he resumed smoking and heavy drinking almost immediately after surgery.

## Illness and treatment - a summary

Half of the patients themselves realised that they had a problem. Many of the remainder had their problem highlighted by their dentist or G.P.

On average, patients stayed in hospital for four weeks. Most of the longer stayers were men. Seventy per cent of the patients stayed in hospital for three weeks or less; more than half stayed between one week and three.

Some patients took longer than others to recover. In this sample, a greater proportion of men than women took more than three weeks - 34 per cent compared to 17 per cent. Some reasons are suggested for this:

-    The men may have presented with more grave conditions in the first place, requiring more time and attention;

-    The men may have been generally in poorer physical condition than the women, and so their systems may have taken longer to get over the physical upheaval;

-    By temperament the women may have been more resilient - they may have been determined to recover more quickly.

Patients found a variety of professionals helpful during hospitalisation, surgeons being the most useful, followed by nurses. Eighteen said that everyone had been helpful, and were not able to be more specific.

## Impact on job and finance

The majority of patients had not worked for many years. Making allowance for the fact that the mean age of the group is around retirement age, this is still high, but it may be due to the high number of patients who were manual workers and who came from Tyneside,

185

Wearside and Teesside, where there has been substantial unemployment for many years. In 1989, for example, when the United Kingdom unemployment level was at 10.6 per cent, unemployment in the northern region was at a level of 14.8 per cent.

Table 7.14 describes when the patients last worked, at the time of first interview.

**Table 7.14**
**When Patient Last Worked    N = 71**
(column percentages in brackets)

Has not worked for:

|  | Male | Female | Total |
|---|---|---|---|
| < 1 month | nil | 1 (4.2) | 1 (1.4) |
| 1 < 3 months | 2 (4.2) | 1 (4.2) | 3 (4.2) |
| 3 < 6 months | 2 (4.2) | 1 (4.2) | 3 (4.2) |
| 6 < 12 months | 3 (6.3) | 1 (4.2) | 4 (5.6) |
| 1 < 2 years | 6 (12.7) | 1 (4.2) | 7 (9.8) |
| 2 years + | 34 (72.3) | 19 (79.2) | 53 (74.6) |
| Total | 47(100.0) | 24(100.0) | 71(100.0) |

Seventy-five per cent of the patients had not worked over the previous two years (this figure includes those who had never worked). More women than men had not worked over the last two years. Of those patients who had worked within the previous two years (25.4%), 27.8 per cent were women, and 72.2 per cent men.

This is not, on the whole, a group of people for whom illness has caused disruption of economic activity; the majority had either never worked, or had not worked for several years. Two thirds of the sample were men, and the mean age for the sample was 63. The picture therefore which prevails is of ageing, working-class men who ceased to be employed, and who subsequently became ill, rather than acute illness and treatment disrupting economic activity - that was only true in a small number of cases.

For a few patients, there were changes in job status. Table 7.15 summarises the patients' job status at the time of the first visit, compared to their status before illness and surgery. Those who had not worked throughout the period have been excluded, leaving 15 men and six women.

## Table 7.15
### Impact on Job (for those economically active)  N = 21
(column percentages in brackets)

| | | |
|---|---|---|
| Promotion | 1 | (4.8) |
| Gained a job | 2 | (9.5) |
| Same job | 12 | (57.1) |
| Similar job | 1 | (4.8) |
| Lost job | 5 | (23.8) |
| | | |
| Total | 21 | 100.0 |

Slightly more men than women had lost jobs since becoming ill, and generally, women were less adversely affected, because fewer of them had been working in the first place.

Five of those who had been economically active had lost their job, and 13 had kept the same or a similar job. So in more cases than not, there was not a negative impact, and indeed a few became employed, and one had been promoted. For a minority, however, there was a deterioration which was ascribable to the illness.

Patients were asked what impact illness and treatment had made on job performance, at the time of first interview, shortly after surgery.

## Table 7.16
### Work Performance  N = 21
(column percentages in brackets)

| | Male | Female | Total |
|---|---|---|---|
| The same | 6 (40.0) | 5 (83.3) | 11 (52.4) |
| Worse | 9 (60.0) | 1 (16.6) | 10 (47.6) |
| | | | |
| Total | 15(100.0) | 6(100.0) | 21(100.0) |

It can be seen that men felt much more adversely affected than women in their work - sixty per cent of men, compared to seventeen per cent of women.

So, for most people, illness and treatment had made little difference to their economic activity; nonetheless, in a small number of instances, there was reduction in income, mainly because of loss of job.

## Variation in income

At first interview, patients were asked what impact illness and treatment had made on income. It was expected to have had a substantial negative impact. Table 7.17 summarises the responses.

**Table 7.17**
**Income Changes    N = 71**
(column percentages in brackets)

|  | Male | Female | Total |
|---|---|---|---|
| Income up | 2  (4.3) | 0 | 2  (2.8) |
| Income the same | 34 (72.3) | 22 (91.7) | 56 (78.9) |
| Income down | 11 (23.4) | 2  (8.3) | 13 (18.3) |
| Total | 47(100.0) | 24(100.0) | 71(100.0) |

In fact, more than three quarters of the patients had no change at all in income. It reduced in 18.3 per cent of cases, and in fact was somewhat higher in two cases.   Of those who had sustained a reduction in income, the greater proportion were men, presumably associated with job loss or absence from work through illness.

This pattern must be set alongside expenditure, and the next table summarises variations in household spending immediately after treatment.

**Table 7.18**
**Changes in Expenditure    N = 71**
(column percentages in brackets)

|  | Male | Female | Total |
|---|---|---|---|
| Expenditure up | 18 (38.3) | 8 (33.3) | 26 (36.6) |
| Expenditure same | 28 (59.6) | 15 (62.5) | 43 (60.6) |
| Expenditure down | 1  (2.1) | 1  (4.2) | 2  (2.8) |
| Total | 47(100.0) | 24(100.0) | 71(100.0) |

The impact on patients and their families was greater in respect of spending than for income. Whereas only 18 per cent had reduced income, 37 per cent had incurred increased expenditure; for just under two thirds, commitments had stayed the same; only two said that they had lower expenditure. The increased expenditure was experienced slightly more by males than by females.

All the increased spending was directly related to illness and treatment. In one instance it was only a temporary increase, although one of the most substantial -this was a patient receiving radiotherapy who paid for taxis to hospital rather than wait for the ambulance. On average, patients spent a further 1.56 pounds per week, with amounts ranging from 0 to 15 pounds. If only the 26 patients who incurred greater expenditure are included in the calculation, they spent on average 4.26 pounds more per week.

Patients were also asked whether there was any change in how they were managing financially. Shortly after surgery, 65 per cent were managing as before, but five women and one man were not managing as well.

### Table 7.19
### Managing Financially    N = 71
(column percentages in brackets)

|         | Male       | Female     | Total      |
|---------|------------|------------|------------|
| Better  | 1  (2.1)   | 2  (8.3)   | 3  (4.2)   |
| The same| 29 (61.7)  | 17 (70.8)  | 46 (64.8)  |
| Worse   | 17 (36.2)  | 5 (20.8)   | 22 (31.0)  |
| Total   | 47(100.0)  | 24(100.0)  | 71(100.0)  |

The majority felt that their capacity to manage money was as good as before, but almost a third felt that their capacity had deteriorated. This may be attributable to the increase in expenditure described above.

### Summary of economic issues

Seventy per cent of the patients were not employed throughout. So for most the illness and treatment had no impact on work, as they were not working anyway.

Thirty per cent of the whole group were either working at the time of becoming ill, or had since got a job. Of these 21 people, more than half had stayed in the same job. Five had lost their job. This was for a number of reasons. For some, the job was unstable anyway. For others, the prolonged illness made it unlikely that they would be fit to return, and in at least one instance, illness caused absence which led to being sacked.

There were only five such people in the study, but they are enough to highlight the vulnerability of those who are working and who sustain oral cancer. At first interview stage it is too early to ask whether facial disfigurement contributed to job loss, but the second interview will consider whether employers found changed appearance unacceptable, and whether the patients themselves felt too self-conscious to go back to work.

More than three quarters of the patients had no change at all in income; eighteen per cent had reduced income, and men were more affected than women. For some, income had gone down because of loss of job. For others, it can be ascribed to their partner's loss of job or reduction in working hours in order to care for their spouse or partner.

Thirty-seven per cent had increased expenditure. All the increased expenditure was directly related to the illness. In all likelihood this would be the same for many serious disorders - use of taxis when the waiting for ambulances could not be tolerated, more heating in the house, more expensive palatable food. Because the increased need was only temporary in many instances, increased benefit would have been difficult to obtain. Where appropriate the interviewer advised or arranged contact with someone who could offer advice on benefits.

## Impact on social life

*Social Contact*

At the outset it had been assumed that people who undergo facial surgery are very isolated people. Patients were therefore asked several questions which addressed this hypothesis. In fact, at the time of first interview no one had not been in social contact with someone in the course of the week prior to the interview, and most had had daily contact, either with the people with whom they were living, with close relatives (such as daughters or sons visiting), or with friends at the pub or club.

As a further indicator of social contact, patients were asked when they had last carried out activities which would necessitate contact with other people. These included shopping and going out to some form of entertainment. Table 7.20 gives details of when individuals last went out shopping.

### Table 7.20
### Shopping     N = 71
(column percentages in brackets)

| Last shopped | Male | Female | Total |
|---|---|---|---|
| Within last week | 15 (31.9) | 5 (20.8) | 20 (28.2) |
| 1 week < 1 month ago | 1 (2.1) | 1 (4.2) | 2 (2.8) |
| 1 < 6 months ago | 7 (15.0) | 2 (8.4) | 9 (12.6) |
| 6 < 12 months ago | 2 (4.2) | 2 (8.4) | 4 (5.6) |
| > 1 year ago | 3 (6.4) | 1 (4.2) | 4 (5.6) |
| Does not normally shop | 19 (40.4) | 13 (54.2) | 32 (45.1) |
| Total | 47(100.0) | 24(100.0) | 71(100.0) |

In a sense, those who did not normally do the shopping (45.1%) were least affected, since they had not gone out for this purpose in the first place. Almost a third of patients resumed going out to shop within a short time (up to one month) from returning from hospital. 23.8 per cent did not appear to have shopped since their recent episode in hospital. Men seemed no slower than women in resuming responsibility for shopping.

In many instances the patients' social life had been minimally interrupted. Patients were asked when they last went out of the house to some form of entertainment. This was interpreted as widely as possible, and responses covered a great variety of activities - for example the local working men's club, dancing club, church groups. Table 7.21 gives details of when the person last left the house to participate in some form of entertainment or leisure activity.

191

## Table 7.21
### Going out to Entertainment    N = 71
(column percentages in brackets)

Last went out to entertainment:

|  | Male | Female | Total |
|---|---|---|---|
| Within the last week | 17 (36.6) | 2 (8.3) | 19 (26.8) |
| 1 < 2 weeks ago | 21 (44.7) | 8 (33.4) | 29 (40.8) |
| 2 weeks < 3 months ago | 3 (6.3) | 8 (33.4) | 11 (15.4) |
| 3 months < 1 year ago | 6 (12.8) | 4 (16.7) | 10 (14.0) |
| 1 < 2 years ago | nil | 1 (4.2) | 1 (1.4) |
| > 2 years ago | nil | 1 (4.2) | 1 (1.4) |
| Total | 47(100.0) | 24(100.0) | 71(100.0) |

The table shows that within the last year almost everyone (97.2 per cent) had been out to some form of leisure or entertainment facility. However, some of this activity would have taken place before surgery. Nonetheless, most patients (67 per cent) had resumed going out to some form of entertainment or leisure, and had gone out within the last week or two. This was true for men more than for women. Several of the men spoken to were keen to resume attendance at the social club or pub as early as possible after discharge; 81.3 per cent had been able to do so, and had been out within the last two weeks.

There was evidence that life was nonetheless more restricted than before. Just over half said that they were unable or less able to carry out leisure and social activities which previously they had enjoyed. It must be remembered that they had only recently undergone substantial surgery, and to a degree one would not necessarily expect any recovering patient to be too outgoing. However, several people said that they had not participated in outside activities precisely because of self-consciousness or because of difficulties in eating or speaking. One lady said that she had enjoyed going out to restaurants with her family, but no longer felt able to do so. Another previously had been part of a church knitting group, and now felt too embarrassed to participate. Some felt diffident about resuming leisure pursuits at this stage, but still hoped to do so before long. The second interview will highlight this.

On the other hand, several patients were interviewed who had resumed social contact immediately; the principal leisure pursuit of several (male) was going out to the club or pub. On the whole they resumed this activity within a few days of leaving hospital. Following on from this, when asked whether there had been any significant change in associating with friends, one third said that there had been. Again, it remains to be seen whether this change is a lasting one.

In order to learn whether surgery and its consequences had caused isolation, the interviewers asked whether patients saw more or less people immediately after treatment than before surgery. Thirty per cent said that they saw less, 68 per cent said that they saw about the same number of people, and only 2.8 per cent (2 people) said that they saw more.

*Social functioning*

Patients commented on levels of functioning in several aspects of their lives, saying whether their functioning in these areas had improved, stayed the same, or had got worse. This is reported in Table 7.22.

### Table 7.22
### Carrying out Home Responsibilities      N = 71
(column percentages in brackets)

|  | Male | Female | Total |
|---|---|---|---|
| Better | 2  (4.3) | 1  (4.2) | 3  (4.2) |
| The same | 22 (46.8) | 12 (50.0) | 34 (47.9) |
| Worse | 23 (48.9) | 11 (45.8) | 34 (47.9) |
| Total | 47(100.0) | 24(100.0) | 71(100.0) |

There is marked deterioration in carrying out home responsibilities - almost half of the patients said that things had got worse in this area. There was little difference between men and women.

When the first interviews were conducted, 43 people lived with a spouse. They were asked whether relations with the spouse had improved, stayed the same, or deteriorated.

## Table 7.23
### Relations with Spouse  N = 43
(column percentages in brackets)

|          | Male       | Female    | Total      |
|----------|------------|-----------|------------|
| Better   | 8 (23.5)   | 3 (33.3)  | 11 (25.6)  |
| The same | 19 (55.9)  | 6 (66.6)  | 25 (58.1)  |
| Worse    | 7 (20.6)   | nil       | 7 (16.3)   |
| Total    | 34(100.0)  | 9(100.0)  | 43(100.0)  |

Some patients got on with their spouse better than previously. They valued more the relationships which they had since their lives had been at risk. For most, however, (58.1%) things had not changed.   For some the situation was worse.

The majority continued to be satisfied with their living environment - house and surroundings.  Details are given in Table 7.24.

## Table 7.24
### Satisfaction with Living Environment  N = 71
(column percentages in brackets)

|          | Male       | Female     | Total      |
|----------|------------|------------|------------|
| More     | 2  (4.3)   | 1  (4.2)   | 3  (4.2)   |
| The same | 39 (83.0)  | 19 (79.2)  | 58 (81.7)  |
| Less     | 6 (12.8)   | 4 (16.7)   | 10 (14.1)  |
| Total    | 47(100.0)  | 24(100.0)  | 71(100.0)  |

There was little or no difference between men and women. There was also little significance in difference in satisfaction with living environment between those for whom there had been a change of household and those for whom there had not. The following table contrasts the position of the seventeen who had moved house with those who did not.

**Table 7.25**
**Change of House and Satisfaction with Living Environment**
**N = 71**

|  | More Satis. | Same | Less Satis. | Total Satis. |
|---|---|---|---|---|
| Change of house | 1 | 13 | 3 | 17 |
| No change of house | 2 | 45 | 7 | 54 |
| Total | 3 | 58 | 10 | 71 |

Finally, there is a substantial group (36.6%) who make less use of community resources such as libraries, parks and swimming pools than previously. 60.6 per cent continued to make as much use as before. The gender distribution is quite even.

**Table 7.26**
**Use of Community Resources     N = 71**
(column percentages in brackets)

|  | Male | Female | Total |
|---|---|---|---|
| More | 1  (2.1) | 1  (4.2) | 2  (2.8) |
| The same | 29 (61.7) | 14 (58.3) | 43 (60.6) |
| Less | 17 (36.2) | 9 (37.5) | 26 (36.6) |
| Total | 47(100.0) | 24(100.0) | 71(100.0) |

Three of the variables addressed above, namely relationship with spouse, carrying out home responsibilities, and use of community resources, were remarkably congruent in their findings. When cross-tabulated with each other, they produced a high level of association, with a high degree of statistical significance. Next, therefore, these three variables were merged to form a new composite variable which represented level of social functioning. A possible score was therefore possible on the new scale of up to nine (three times the maximum score of three for each of the original three variables). Scores from three to six were described as low, and scores from seven to nine were described as high. Cross-tabulations were then carried out with a number of variables in order to see which of them influenced social functioning.

First, the influence of age on social functioning was considered. Table 7.27 summarises the results.

### Table 7.27
### Age and Social Functioning     N = 71
(row percentages in brackets)

| Social Functioning | Low | High | Total |
|---|---|---|---|
| Age | | | |
| 30 < 40 | 3 (60.0) | 2 (40.0) | 5 |
| 40 < 50 | 6 (75.0) | 2 (25.0) | 8 |
| 50 < 60 | 5 (33.3) | 10 (66.7) | 15 |
| 60 < 70 | 7 (36.8) | 12 (63.2) | 15 |
| 70 < 80 | 8 (44.4) | 10 (55.6) | 18 |
| 80 + | 3 (50.0) | 3 (50.0) | 6 |
| Total | 32 (45.1) | 39 (54.9) | 71 |

The results were slightly short of acceptable probability (chi squared = 44.8, p = .08), but some trends can be seen. Broadly, those up to the age of 50 functioned better than those aged 50 to 80. Those aged 80 and above fared slightly better.

Next, gender was considered in relation to social functioning. Table 7.28 summarises the results.

### Table 7.28
### Gender and Social Functioning     N = 71
(row percentages in brackets)

| Social Functioning | Low | High | Total |
|---|---|---|---|
| Gender | | | |
| Male | 20 (42.5) | 27 (57.4) | 47 |

196

'continued'

| | | | |
|---|---|---|---|
| Female | 12 (50.0) | 12 (50.0) | 24 |
| Total | 32 (45.1) | 39 (54.9) | 71 |

The results were not significant. Acknowledging this, it can be seen that a greater proportion of men functioned in the higher range than women.

The influence of area of residence was next related to social functioning - what type of area, urban, suburban and rural.

**Table 7.29**
**Area and Social Functioning   N = 71**
(row percentages in brackets)

Social Functioning

| Area | Low | High | Total |
|---|---|---|---|
| Urban | 7 (35.0) | 13 (65.0) | 20 |
| Suburban | 18 (43.9) | 23 (56.1) | 41 |
| Rural | 7 (70.0) | 3 (30.0) | 10 |
| Total | 32 (45.1) | 39 (54.9) | 71 |

The results did not reach a significant level. Nonetheless, a clear trend exists within the sample, whereby urban dwellers functioned higher than suburban, and both functioned substantially higher than country dwellers.

Most of those interviewed either lived alone or with their spouse. Only seven had any living arrangement different from this. Looking only at the 64 who either lived with a spouse or lived alone, Table 7.30 considered the impact of living situation on social functioning.

## Table 7.30
### Living Situation and Social Functioning    N = 71
(row percentages in brackets)

Social Functioning

| Living Situation | Low | High | Total |
|---|---|---|---|
| With Spouse | 17 (39.5) | 26 (60.5) | 43 |
| Alone | 11 (52.4) | 10 (47.6) | 21 |
| Total | 28 (43.7) | 36 (56.2) | 64 |

The results were not significant. They suggested that those living with a spouse were functioning somewhat better than those who lived alone.

The association between social class and social functioning was examined. The results are summarised in Table 7.31.

## Table 7.31
### Social Class and Social Functioning    N = 71
(row percentages in brackets)

Social Functioning

| | Low | High | Total |
|---|---|---|---|
| White Collar | 3 (30.0) | 7 (70.0) | 10 |
| Manual | 29 (47.5) | 32 (52.5) | 61 |
| Total | 32 (45.1) | 39 (54.9) | 71 |

The results were not significant. It can be seen that patients with non-manual background were functioning better than those of manual background.

It has already been reported that patients were asked whether the original (excising) surgery had been successful, in the sense of eradicating the tumour. Their responses were considered in association with their social functioning, and reported in Table 7.32.

### Table 7.32
### Outcome of Surgery and Social Functioning    N = 71
(row percentages in brackets)

Social Functioning

| Outcome | Low | High | Total |
|---|---|---|---|
| Successful | 24 (48.0) | 26 (52.0) | 50 |
| Not Successful | 5 (83.3) | 1 (16.7) | 6 |
| Not Sure | 3 (20.0) | 12 (80.0) | 15 |
| Total | 32 (45.1) | 39 (54.9) | 71 |

The results were highly significant (chi squared = 37.8 at probability level of .00056). Those who considered that outcome had been successful were reported to be functioning at a substantially higher level than those who felt that surgery had not been successful. Curiously, those who were unsure about the successful outcome of surgery were functioning highest of all.

Patients had been asked whether they felt better or worse in themselves than before illness and treatment. Table 7.33 describes the relationship between the responses and social functioning.

### Table 7.33
### Current Feeling and Social Functioning    N = 71
(row percentages in brackets)

Social Functioning

| Feeling | Low | High | Total |
|---|---|---|---|
| Better | 8 (47.1) | 9 (52.9) | 17 |
| The same | 14 (66.7) | 7 (33.3) | 21 |
| Worse | 10 (30.3) | 23 (69.7) | 33 |
| Total | 32 (45.1) | 39 (54.9) | 71 |

The results were not significant. Those who said that they were feeling the same were functioning at a lower level. Those who were feeling better were fairly evenly distributed, while those who were feeling worse were in fact functioning better.

Finally, in this consideration of influences on social functioning, the patient's outlook on life was related to social functioning. How a view on the patient's outlook was achieved is described below; suffice to say that it represented a composite of several features which together could confidently be seen as a measure of their view of themselves in relation to life and the world. Table 7.34 describes the relationship between the two variables, outlook and social functioning.

**Table 7.34**
**Outlook and Social Functioning     N = 71**
(row percentages in brackets)

Social Functioning

| Outlook | Low | High | Total |
|---|---|---|---|
| Low | 2 (16.6) | 10 (83.3) | 12 |
| Medium | 17 (45.9) | 20 (54.1) | 37 |
| High | 13 (59.1) | 9 (40.9) | 22 |
| Total | 32 (45.1) | 39 (54.9) | 71 |

The results were significant - chi squared $= 9.6$ at a probability level of .04690. A very clear association can be seen between outlook and functioning. Those whose outlook was poor also functioned at a low level. Those whose outlook was more positive - either medium or high - were more evenly distributed between low and high social functioning scores.

## Outlook

Next, patients were asked to comment on their overall mood and outlook, by saying how enthusiastic they felt about life, how fulfilled they felt in their life, and how optimistic they felt about the future. They were asked to note each area at a point on a five point scale, from enthusiastic to apathetic, from fulfilled to unfulfilled, and from optimistic to pessimistic. When they were unsure about the meaning of the terms, they were expressed to them in an alternative, more understandable way. The responses are only impressions, taken on a certain day, when patients were feeling a certain way. They are intended only as an additional insight into the functioning of the patients in the study.

The first such indicator refers to the level of enthusiasm which patients felt about life. Table 7.35 describes their responses.

**Table 7.35**
**Level of Enthusiasm for Life     N = 71**
(column percentages in brackets)

|  | Male | Female | Total |
|---|---|---|---|
| Enthusiastic | 7 (14.9) | 2 (8.3) | 9 (12.7) |
| 4. | 8 (17.0) | 5 (20.8) | 13 (18.3) |
| 3. | 15 (31.9) | 10 (41.7) | 25 (35.2) |
| 2. | 14 (29.8) | 6 (25.0) | 20 (28.2) |
| Apathetic | 3 (6.4) | 1 (4.2) | 4 (5.6) |
| Total | 47(100.0) | 24(100.0) | 71(100.0) |

Responses were fairly evenly distributed - a third enthusiastic and a third apathetic about life.

The question in relation to self-fulfilment was explained to patients in terms of how much they had achieved in relation to their ambitions. Inevitably, this means different things to people depending on their age.

## Table 7.36
### Level of Fulfilment    N = 71
(column percentages in brackets)

|  | Male | Female | Total |
|---|---|---|---|
| Fulfilled | 5 (10.6) | 3 (12.5) | 8 (11.3) |
| 4. | 9 (19.1) | 4 (16.7) | 13 (18.3) |
| 3. | 16 (34.0) | 13 (54.2) | 29 (40.8) |
| 2. | 13 (27.7) | 1 (4.2) | 14 (19.7) |
| Missed Chances | 4 (8.5) | 3 (12.5) | 7 (9.9) |
| Total | 47(100.0) | 24(100.0) | 71(100.0) |

Responses on fulfilment were evenly distributed. Women's responses tended to gather round the mid-point more than those of the men, who regarded themselves as slightly less fulfilled overall than the women.

## Table 7.37
### Level of Optimism    N = 71
(column percentages in brackets)

|  | Male | Female | Total |
|---|---|---|---|
| Optimistic | 7 (14.9) | 3 (12.5) | 10 (14.1) |
| 4. | 8 (17.0) | 3 (12.5) | 11 (15.5) |
| 3. | 10 (21.3) | 10 (41.7) | 20 (28.2) |
| 2. | 14 (29.8) | 6 (25.0) | 20 (28.2) |
| Pessimistic | 8 (17.O) | 2 (8.3) | 10 (14.1) |
| Total | 47(100.0) | 24(100.0) | 71(100.0) |

Men tended to be more pessimistic than women, and generally, there was a tendency to pessimism.

It can be seen that very similar results were obtained for each of these three questions. In order to achieve a more robust scale or measure of outlook, the three variables were then merged. First, the results for each were compared with the rest, to ensure that the questions were addressing broadly the same area of concern. What emerged was that there was a high degree of association between each of three variables, and a very high level of significance.

The three variables were therefore merged, thus producing a 15-point scale (the sum of the scores for each of three variables, each of which had possible score of five). Generally, the results on this scale are summarised as "low, medium and high", in order to overcome the difficulty of low scores in the cells of the tables.

The new composite variable "Outlook" was then considered in relation to a number of descriptive variables, in order to see whether any of them could be seen to have influenced patient outlook.

The first of these was age. Table 7.38 describes the association between age and outlook. The results were not significant.

### Table 7.38
### Age and Outlook    N = 71

Outlook

| Age | Low | Medium | High | Total |
|---|---|---|---|---|
| 30 < 40 | 1 | 1 | 3 | 5 |
| 40 < 50 | 2 | 4 | 2 | 8 |
| 50 < 60 | 6 | 6 | 3 | 15 |
| 60 < 70 | 3 | 11 | 5 | 19 |
| 70 < 80 | nil | 11 | 7 | 18 |
| 80 + | nil | 4 | 2 | 6 |
| Total | 12 | 37 | 22 | 71 |

Although the scores were not significant, they were approaching significance - chi squared = 13.7 at a probability level of .18467.

Percentages have not been calculated, because of the small scores in most cells. Little overall pattern is evident, but remembering that outlook scores overall are in the proportion 1:3:2 of the low:medium:high distribution, it can be seen that no one age group actually fits this proportion. Those in their thirties to sixties tend to score lower, while those over 70 score disproportionately high.

Next, the relationship of gender to outlook was examined. A

summary of the distribution is given in Table 7.39. The results did not achieve significance.

### Table 7.39
### Gender and Outlook   N = 71
(row percentages in brackets)

|  | Low | Medium | High | Total |
|---|---|---|---|---|
| **Gender** | | | | |
| Male | 9 (19.1) | 23 (48.9) | 15 (31.9) | 47 |
| Female | 3 (12.5) | 14 (58.3) | 7 (29.2) | 24 |
| Total | 12 (31.6) | 37(52.1) | 22 (31.0) | 71 |

Outlook appeared slightly influenced by gender. A greater proportion of women than men had medium scores for outlook, while more men had both high and low scores.

Most of those interviewed either lived alone or lived with a spouse - 43 with a spouse and 21 alone. The mean outlook on the fifteen point scale for those living with a spouse was 8.2, and for those living alone 9.1. The following table further illustrates the point that those living alone had a better outlook on life than those living with a spouse.

### Table 7.40
### Living Situation and Outlook   N = 71
(row percentages in brackets)

|  | Low | Medium | High | Total |
|---|---|---|---|---|
| With Spouse | 7 (16.3) | 22 (51.2) | 14 (32.6) | 43 |
| Alone | 2 (9.5) | 11 (52.4) | 8 (38.1) | 21 |
| Total | 12 (16.9) | 37 (52.1) | 22 (31.0) | 71 |

Those living alone tended to score slightly higher than those living with a spouse. Overall, around half of those interviewed gave a response in the middle range, but fewer patients living with a spouse scored high. Statistical significance was not achieved.

The effect of social class on outlook was then considered. The results are given in Table 7.41. In order to give a clearer summary of the trends, the categories of social class have been simplified into "white collar" and "manual". Those who were not classified have been grouped with manual, since, as was stated earlier, this represented the estimate of the interviewer of their social status.

### Table 7.41
### Social Class and Outlook    N = 71
(row percentages in brackets)

|              | Low        | Medium      | High        | Total |
| ------------ | ---------- | ----------- | ----------- | ----- |
| White Collar | 1 (10.0)   | 2 (20.0)    | 7 (70.0)    | 10    |
| Manual       | 11 (18.0)  | 35 (57.4)   | 15 (24.6)   | 61    |
| Total        | 12 (16.9)  | 37 (52.1)   | 22 (31.0)   | 71    |

The results were highly significant - chi squared = 8.3 at a probability level of .01583. They suggested that the outlook of white collar workers was substantially more positive than that of manual workers, most of whose responses fell into the middle range.

### Summary of social consequences

All of the patients were in contact at least weekly with relatives, friends or neighbours. Most had daily contact with someone. So, none of the patients in the study was completely isolated: everyone was in touch with someone at least once a week, and 50 out of the 71 lived with someone else anyway. However, there were indicators that life had become more restricted. Twenty-four per cent had not shopped in the last six months, and 33 per cent had not resumed their previous leisure activities. Forty-eight per cent reported a lessening of their ability to carry out home responsibilities, with little difference between men and women.

However, as the surgeons consistently stress, it takes many months before life is resumed in its entirety - before eating becomes easy and enjoyable, before full arm movement becomes pain-free, before feelings of nausea fade, and before speech becomes intelligible and without self-consciousness. For some there is always a residue, but the point here is that it would be surprising if normal activities had been completely resumed. The crucial test is whether such restriction has persisted at the end of a further year.

Social functioning was influenced by a number of social factors:

- age - those aged up to fifty fared better than those over fifty;

- gender - men functioned better than women;

- area - those who lived in towns functioned more successfully than those who lived in the country;

- household composition - those who lived with someone else functioned better than those who lived alone;

- patients with a non-manual occupation background functioned better than manual workers;

- if patients felt that surgery had been successful, they tended to be functioning better. This result was highly significant;

- sense of well-being bore little relation to actual social functioning;

- there was a positive association between outlook and social functioning.

When questions about outlook were introduced into the interview schedule, it was not with the intention of conducting a complete psychological appraisal, but rather to obtain a quick overview. Responses to the question about enthusiasm for life were evenly distributed - one third enthusiastic, one third moderate, and one third apathetic. A similar distribution was obtained in response to the question on fulfilment. The question on level of optimism produced somewhat more negative results - 42.3 per cent were tending towards pessimism.

The effect of other social factors on outlook was considered. This is summarised as follows:

- those aged up to seventy tended to have poorer outlook than those over seventy;

- women tended to have moderate outlook scores, while men tended more towards the two extremes;

- the outlook of those living alone was slightly better than that of those living with someone else;

- white collar workers scored substantially (and significantly) higher for outlook than manual workers.


**Facial appearance**

No objective measure of appearance was undertaken in this study. It must be remembered that this was an attempt to obtain patients' viewpoints, and so what mattered in this respect was their satisfaction with their appearance, past and present. As far as could be gauged, satisfaction with appearance did not seem to be related to the extent of the surgery. For example, one woman who had an intra-oral scar felt severely disfigured, whereas a man with a large abdominal flap covering the greater part of one side of his face felt in no way disfigured.

Immediately after surgery, participants were asked to say whether they were satisfied with their past appearance, and their responses were placed on a five-point scale, ranging from "complete contentment" to "hating their appearance".

They were then asked to say how satisfied they were with their present appearance after surgery, and the same five-point scale was used to chart their responses.

The two sets of responses are reproduced in graph form in Table 7.42. Please see following page.

**Table 7.42**
**Satisfaction with Appearance - Past and Present  N = 71**

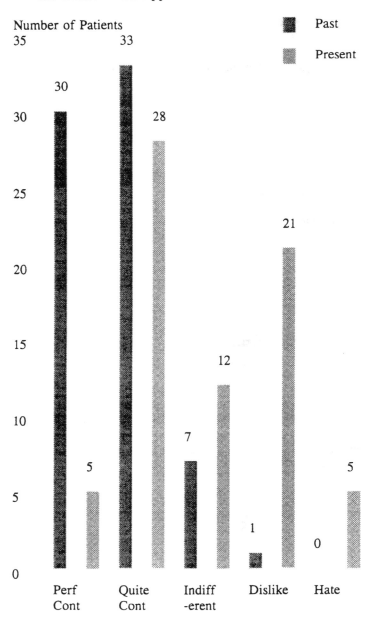

Most patients rated themselves as "perfectly content" or "quite content" with their past appearance. Only one person was found to have disliked their past appearance, and nobody "hated" it. Satisfaction with present appearance was substantially less. 54 per cent of women now disliked or hated their appearance, and 28 per cent of men.

Nobody rated their appearance as better than past appearance. The differences between the two ratings are summarised in Table 7.43.

**Table 7.43**
**Difference in Satisfaction with Past and Present Appearance**
**N = 71**
(column percentages in brackets)

|  | Male | Female | Total |
|---|---|---|---|
| No different | 20 (42.5) | 7 (29.1) | 27 (38.0) |
| 1 point lower | 13 (27.6) | 6 (25.0) | 19 (26.8) |
| 2 points lower | 7 (14.9) | 5 (20.8) | 12 (16.9) |
| 3 points lower | 6 (12.8) | 4 (16.7) | 10 (14.1) |
| 4 points lower | 1 (2.1) | 2 (8.3) | 3 (4.2) |
| Total | 47(100.0) | 24(100.0) | 71(100.0) |

This information must be treated with caution: patients were only just recovering from surgery at this stage, and their appearance, together with their satisfaction about it, could be expected to improve over the next few months. Secondly, the fact that patients disliked their present appearance does not mean that they would not have wanted to go through surgery, as the principal reason for the surgery was to save their lives. In addition, patients could well be remembering with something of a halo effect their appearance before illness.

Next, these differences between satisfaction with previous appearance and satisfaction with present appearance were set alongside certain variables, to see if there was any association between change in satisfaction and other external variables. First, age of patients was considered. Table 7.44 gives the results. Percentages have not been provided, because of the low scores in each cell.

**Table 7.44**

**Table 7.44**
### Age and Change in Satisfaction with Appearance  N = 71

Satisfaction with appearance

| Age | Same | 1 Pt Lower | 2 Pts Lower | 3 Pts Lower | 4 Pts | Total |
|---|---|---|---|---|---|---|
| 30 < 40 | 2 | 1 | 1 | 1 | nil | 5 |
| 40 < 50 | 3 | 2 | 2 | 1 | nil | 8 |
| 50 < 60 | 7 | 4 | 2 | 1 | 1 | 15 |
| 60 < 70 | 7 | 2 | 4 | 5 | 1 | 19 |
| 70 < 80 | 6 | 7 | 2 | 2 | 1 | 18 |
| 80+ | 2 | 3 | 1 | nil | nil | 6 |
| Total | 27 | 19 | 12 | 10 | 3 | 71 |

Because of the fact that the results were not significant, and because of the small numbers in each of the cells, interpretation is difficult, but it can be seen that the exception to the pattern is for those in their sixties, where most of the 19 have reduced their satisfaction with appearance, and several markedly so.

Gender differences were then considered. Again, the results were not significant, and they are summarised in Table 7.45.

**Table 7.45**
### Gender and Change in Satisfaction with Appearance N = 64
(row percentages in brackets)

Satisfaction with appearance

| Gender | Same | 1 Pt Lower | 2 Pts Lower | 3 Pts Lower | 4 Pts Lower | Total |
|---|---|---|---|---|---|---|
| Male | 20 (42.5) | 13 (27.7) | 7 (14.9) | 6 (12.8) | 1 (2.1) | 47 (100.0) |
| Female | 7 (29.2) | 6 (25.0) | 5 (20.8) | 4 (16.7) | 2 (8.3) | 24 (100.0) |

'continued'

Total  23     18     12     8      3      64
       (35.9) (28.1) (18.7) (12.5) (4.7) (100.0)


A greater proportion of men than women reported no change in satisfaction with their appearance - 42 per cent compared to 29 per cent. More men reported one point difference, and for two, three and four points different women were the larger proportion. The association between living situation and changed satisfaction with appearance was then considered. Since most of those interviewed (64) either lived with spouse or lived alone other situations were excluded, in order to obtain a clearer contrast. Table 7.46 gives the results.


**Table 7.46**
**Living Situation and Change in Satisfaction with Appearance**
**N = 64**
(row percentages in brackets)

Satisfaction with appearance

|  | Same | 1 Pt Lower | 2 Pts Lower | 3 Pts Lower | 4 Pts Lower | Total |
|---|---|---|---|---|---|---|
| Living situation | | | | | | |
| Spouse | 20 | 9 | 7 | 4 | 3 | 43 |
|  | (46.5) | (20.9) | (16.3) | (9.3) | (7.0) | (100.0) |
| Alone | 3 | 9 | 5 | 4 | nil | 21 |
|  | (14.3) | (42.9) | (23.8) | (19.0) |  | (100.0) |
| Total | 23 | 18 | 12 | 8 | 3 | 64 |
|  | (35.9) | (28.1) | (18.7) | (12.5) | (4.7) | (100.0) |


The results were not significant. Those who lived alone reported slightly more reduction in satisfaction with appearance than those who lived with a spouse.

Social class was then considered. The social class categories were simplified into manual and non-manual. Table 7.47 describes the results.

## Table 7.47
## Social Class and Change in Satisfaction with Appearance
## N = 71
(row percentages in brackets)

Satisfaction with appearance

|  | Same | 1 Pt Lower | 2 Pts Lower | 3 Pts Lower | 4 Pts Lower | Total |
|---|---|---|---|---|---|---|
| Non-manual | 3 (30.0) | 4 (40.0) | 2 (20.0) | 1 (10.0) | nil | 10 (100.0) |
| Manual | 24 (39.3) | 15 (24.6) | 10 (16.4) | 9 (14.7) | 3 (4.9) | 61 (100.0) |
| Total | 27 (38.0) | 19 (26.8) | 12 (16.9) | 10 (14.1) | 3 (4.2) | 71 (100.0) |

There were only 10 non-manual patients interviewed, and so it is hard to rely on the results, which were not statistically significant. No clear pattern emerged from the analysis, and on the face of it it must be concluded that social class did not influence change in satisfaction with appearance.

Whether the patient viewed the outcome of surgery was considered in relation to change in satisfaction with appearance. Table 7.48 describes the results.

## Table 7.48
## Outcome of Surgery and Change in Satisfaction with Appearance    N = 71
(row percentages in brackets)

Satisfaction with appearance

|  | Same | 1 Pt Lower | 2 Pts Lower | 3 Pts Lower | 4 Pts Lower | Total |
|---|---|---|---|---|---|---|
| Success? |  |  |  |  |  |  |
| Yes | 18 (36.0) | 16 (32.0) | 8 (16.0) | 6 (12.0) | 2 (4.0) | 50 (100.0) |

'continued'

| | Same | 1 Pt Lower | 2 Pts Lower | 3 Pts Lower | 4 Pts Lower | Total |
|---|---|---|---|---|---|---|
| No | 4 | nil | 1 | 1 | nil | 6 |
| | (39.3) | (24.6) | (16.4) | (14.7) | (4.9) | (100.0) |
| Not sure | 5 | 3 | 3 | 3 | 1 | 15 |
| | (33.3) | (20.0) | (20.0) | (20.0) | (6.7) | (100.0) |
| Total | 27 | 19 | 12 | 10 | 3 | 71 |
| | (38.0) | (26.8) | (16.9) | (14.1) | (4.2) | (100.0) |

The results were not significant. There was virtually no difference in changed satisfaction between those who believed that surgical outcome was successful and those who felt that it was not. Those who were unsure whether outcome had been successful were slightly more likely to have changed for the worse their level of satisfaction with their appearance.

Patients had also been asked if they felt generally better or worse than before surgery. The results were now correlated with their comments on changed satisfaction with appearance. This is described in Table 7.49.

**Table 7.49**
**Current Well-being and Change in Satisfaction with Appearance**
**N = 71**
(row percentages in brackets)

Satisfaction with appearance

| | Same | 1 Pt Lower | 2 Pts Lower | 3 Pts Lower | 4 Pts Lower | Total |
|---|---|---|---|---|---|---|
| Feeling better | 7 | 6 | 2 | 2 | nil | 17 |
| | (41.2) | (35.3) | (11.8) | (11.8) | | (100.0) |
| Same | 11 | 6 | 2 | 1 | 1 | 21 |
| | (39.3) | (24.6) | (16.4) | (14.7) | (4.9) | (100.0) |
| Worse | 9 | 7 | 8 | 7 | 2 | 33 |
| | (27.3) | (21.2) | (24.2) | (21.2) | (6.1) | (100.0) |
| Total | 27 | 19 | 12 | 10 | 3 | 71 |
| | (38.0) | (26.8) | (16.9) | (14.1) | (4.2) | (100.0) |

Although the results were not significant, it emerged that those who felt better were also more content with their appearance.

Those who saw more people might be seen not to have changed their view of their appearance as much as those who saw less. In fact, only two patients had seen more than before. The chief distinction lay between those who had seen less people and those who had seen the same number. This analysis is described in Table 7.50.

**Table 7.50**
**People Seen and Change in Satisfaction with Appearance**
**N = 71**
(row percentages in brackets)

Satisfaction with appearance

|  | Same | 1 Pt Lower | 2 Pts Lower | 3 Pts Lower | 4 Pts Lower | Total |
|---|---|---|---|---|---|---|
| Less People | 7 (33.3) | 2 (9.5) | 5 (23.8) | 4 (19.0) | 3 (14.3) | 21 (100.0) |
| Same Number | 19 (39.6) | 17 (35.4) | 6 (12.5) | 6 (12.5) | nil | 48 (100.0) |
| More People | 1 (50.0) | nil | 1 (50.0) | nil | nil | 2 (100.0) |
| Total | 27 (38.0) | 19 (26.8) | 12 (16.9) | 10 (14.1) | 3 (4.2) | 71 (100.0) |

Those who saw fewer people tended to have changed their satisfaction with their appearance for the worse. The results were verging on significance - chi squared = 14.7 at a probability level of .06408.

The composite variable Outlook was then correlated with changed in satisfaction with appearance, and was found to be very significant - chi-squared = 18.9 at a probability level of .01522. The results are given in Table 7.51.

Table 7.51

**Outlook and Change in Satisfaction with Appearance**  N = 71
(row percentages in brackets)
Satisfaction with appearance

| Outlook | Same | 1 Pt Lower | 2 Pts Lower | 3 Pts Lower | 4 Pts Lower | Total |
|---|---|---|---|---|---|---|
| Poor | 4 | nil | 2 | 5 | 1 | 12 |
| | (33.3) | | (16.7) | (41.7) | (8.3) | (100.0) |
| Medium | 17 | 8 | 7 | 3 | 2 | 37 |
| | (45.9) | (21.6) | (18.9) | (8.1) | (5.4) | (100.0) |
| High | 6 | 11 | 3 | 2 | nil | 22 |
| | (27.3) | (50.0) | (13.6) | (9.1) | | (100.0) |
| Total | 27 | 19 | 12 | 10 | 3 | 71 |
| | (38.0) | (26.8) | (16.9) | (14.1) | (4.2) | (100.0) |

Two thirds of those whose outlook on life was reported as low tended to have changed for the worse their level of satisfaction with their appearance. The most stable group was those whose outlook was moderate - 45 per cent had not changed at all, and a further 21 per cent had only changed to one point lower. Those with the highest expectations of life tended to have experienced little or no change in satisfaction with appearance - 77 per cent had changed only one point or not at all.

At first interview, many felt that people had changed in their attitude to them since surgery. This was usually described by saying that people stared at them more and made them more self-conscious. Details are given in Table 7.52.

**Table 7.52**
**Changes in People's Attitude to Patient**  N = 71

| | Male % | Female % | Total % |
|---|---|---|---|
| Yes | 23 (48.9) | 16 (66.7) | 39 (54.9) |
| No | 24 (51) | 8 (33.3) | 32 (45.1) |
| Total | 47 (100.0) | 24 (100.0) | 71 (100.0) |

More women than men felt that others had changed in their attitude to them, but the overall felt difference was 54.9%. A year later, fewer people felt that people had changed in their attitude to them as a result of illness and surgery, only 46.2%. This was despite the fact that 75.0% felt that their appearance had altered as a result of surgery.

This profile of change of attitudes was considered as a possible influence on patients' changed acceptance of their appearance. Table 7.53 describes the results of this analysis. The results were not statistically significant.

### Table 7.53
### Attitude of Others and Change in Satisfaction with Appearance
### N = 71
(row percentages in brackets)

Satisfaction with appearance

People changed attitudes?

|       | Same | 1 Pt Lower | 2 Pts Lower | 3 Pts Lower | 4 Pts Lower | Total |
|-------|------|------------|-------------|-------------|-------------|-------|
| Yes   | 11   | 10         | 8           | 8           | 2           | 39    |
|       | (28.2) | (25.6)   | (20.5)      | (20.5)      | (5.1)       | (100.0) |
| No    | 16   | 9          | 4           | 2           | 1           | 32    |
|       | (50.0) | (28.1)   | (12.5)      | (6.2)       | (3.1)       | (100.0) |
| Total | 27   | 19         | 12          | 10          | 3           | 71    |
|       | (38.0) | (26.8)   | (16.9)      | (14.1)      | (4.2)       | (100.0) |

Where people were thought by patients to have changed their attitude to them since surgery, the patients too were less accepting of their appearance than before surgery.

### Summary

Satisfaction with present appearance was substantially less than with past appearance. Those in their sixties reported the greatest reduction in satisfaction with appearance, and more women than men disliked

216

their present appearance. In addition, more women than men felt that others had changed in their attitudes to them. Social class did not appear to influence change in satisfaction, and neither to any great extent did household composition.

## Conclusion

The empirical study was designed to test 16 hypotheses. These are outlined in Chapter Seven, and they will be examined in Chapter Eleven, in the light of the experience of the two sets of interviews. However, at this stage the following preliminary observations are made. The group interviewed was composed mostly of working-class, ageing men. This is consistent with the literature on head and neck cancer. The social profile of the group will also have a bearing on the survival rate, which will be discussed in the next chapter.

Men reacted to illness and treatment differently from women: women expressed earlier concern about their condition, while men appeared to deny its existence for some time. Men stayed in hospital longer than women.

The importance of primary dental care was highlighted by the frequency with which the dental practitioner discovered the presence of a malignancy.

Most people in the group were not wage-earning (The extent of dependency on state benefits will be discussed in Chapter Ten). This is one aspect of the pattern of powerlessness which is evident in the group: the members have few choices, and their power is restricted by their low income. This in turn affected their outlook on life, which was less positive for manual workers than for white collar workers.

Those interviewed were not entirely cut off from other people, but their lives were more restricted than before illness. They were less able to participate in leisure activities, and some were not able to get out to shop. This could well be due to the fact that they were recovering from illness and major surgery; it is premature to ascribe it to disfigurement.

At this early stage, those who were functioning better were younger, male, living in towns, with someone else in their household. They were of non-manual background, with a positive outlook on life.

For every one of the patients interviewed, treatment resulted in mutilation, although for many the visible effects of this mutilation diminished before they were seen again by the research interviewer. While remembering that the study only takes account of a patient's view of their appearance, at the same time it is the patient's view of his or her own appearance in this context that matters. The views of patients a year later are even more crucial, when healing has been allowed to be completed. Meanwhile, the results are sobering. No doubt most patients would accept the disfigurement, felt or real, as the price for survival, but nonetheless at this early stage more than half the patients disliked or hated the visible results of the surgical procedure.

Surgeons were felt to be helpful, not only as clinicians, but also as communicators and counsellors. Nurses too were appreciated by many of those interviewed. Few other professionals were seen as helpful; this is cause for concern: first, because patients felt the lack of help, particularly after they had returned home, and secondly because several professionals who see it as their role to respond to the needs of ill and recovering people did not do so: social workers, chaplains, general medical practitioners, health visitors. People have been in need, while professionals who might have met that need have failed to do so. This tragic gap, and suggestions for reducing it, will be discussed in the concluding chapter.

In this chapter the emphasis has been on acute illness and surgery. In the next two chapters a different focus will be presented: the extent of recovery and resumption of normal life. A proportion of people did not recover, and so one of the issues which will be addressed is survival itself. In Chapter Eleven, the lessons derived from both sets of interviews will be used in order to test out the hypotheses on which the study is based.

# 8 Survival

Ildstad et al.[1] considered the possible characteristics which influence the survival of patients with head and neck cancer, by means of a regression analysis of 542 patients. The factor which most influenced survival was the tumour stage at the point of presentation. Advanced age and location of the tumour in the tonsillar area were also associated with poor survival. Type of therapy and gender were not significant. So, if the patients was old, had a tumour around the tonsillar area, and did not go for treatment until the tumour was well advanced, the survival chances were lowest.

In this chapter influences on survival are considered, but unlike Ilstadt et al., I shall consider only social influences. None of the associations described reached statistical significance. It therefore remains open to question whether the results are representative of the wider population.

It will be remembered that 53 of the original group of 71 were still alive at the time of the second interview - 74.6 per cent survived, 25.4 per cent did not.

The rate of survival for each age group is considered in Table 8.1.

**Table 8.1**
**Age and Survival     N = 71**
(row percentages in brackets)

|         | Survived   | Died      | Total |
|---------|------------|-----------|-------|
| 30 < 40 | 5(100.0)   | 0         | 5     |
| 40 < 50 | 5 (62.5)   | 3 (37.5)  | 8     |
| 50 < 60 | 11 (73.3)  | 4 (26.7)  | 15    |
| 60 < 70 | 13 (68.4)  | 6 (31.6)  | 19    |

219

'continued'

| | | | |
|---|---|---|---|
| 70 < 80 | 14 (77.8) | 4 (22.2) | 18 |
| 80+ | 5 (83.3) | 1 (16.7) | 6 |
| Total | 53 (74.6) | 18 (25.4) | 71 (100.0) |

Strong inferences cannot be drawn from such small numbers, but in this group, the age group with the second highest survival rate was the oldest age group. Those in their thirties had all survived, while the highest mortality was in those in their forties, followed by those in their sixties, and then those in their fifties. Those in their seventies, who were present in reasonably large numbers, survived almost as well as those in their eighties. Thus, a different pattern has been established from that suggested by Ilstadt, who said that advancing age was an indicator for mortality in head and neck tumours.

The proportions of each gender who survived are described in Table 8.2.

### Table 8.2
### Gender and Survival    N = 71
(row percentages in brackets)

| | Survived | Died | Total |
|---|---|---|---|
| Male | 33 (70.2) | 14 (29.8) | 47(100.0) |
| Female | 20 (83.3) | 4 (16.7) | 24(100.0) |
| Total | 53 (74.6) | 18 (25.4) | 71(100.0) |

Remembering that the results were not significant, it can still be seen that a noticeably higher proportion of men than women died.

There were strong differences between the survival rates of the social class groups. Details are given in Table 8.3.

### Table 8.3
### Social Class and Survival  N = 71
(row percentages in brackets)

|  | Survived | Not Survived | Total |
|---|---|---|---|
| White Collar | 9 (90.0) | 1 (10.0) | 10 (100.0) |
| Manual | 44 (69.6) | 17 (30.4) | 61 (100.0) |
| Total | 53 (74.6) | 18 (25.4) | 71(100.0) |

By the time of the second interviews, 90% of the white collar group were still alive, compared to 69.6% of the manual workers. 80% of the unclassified (women) had survived.

Where the patient lived - whether in town or country - had a strong association with survival. Table 8.4 describes the original living situation of the patients, and whether they survived.

### Table 8.4
### Area of Residence (at First Interview) and Survival
### N = 71
(row percentages in brackets)

|  | Survived | Not Survived | Total |
|---|---|---|---|
| Urban | 12 (60.0) | 8 (40.0) | 20(100.0) |
| Suburban | 33 (80.5) | 8 (19.5) | 41(100.0) |
| Rural | 8 (80.0) | 2 (20.0) | 10(100.0) |
| Total | 53 (74.6) | 18 (25.4) | 71(100.0) |

Forty per cent of urban dwellers had died by the time of the second interview, compared to 19 per cent of suburban dwellers, and 20 percent of those who lived in the country. Despite the lack of statistical significance (chi squared = 6.2 at a probability level of .18665), the trend cannot be ignored; those who lived in the towns and cities sustained twice the mortality rate of those who lived outside town and city centres.

Table 8.5 describes the proportions of survivors according to the person(s) with whom they lived. For this purpose, only the first named person with whom each lived has been used. Since the numbers of those who lived with anyone other than a spouse were very small, they have been excluded from this table, in order to accentuate the contrast between those who lived alone and those who lived with a spouse.

**Table 8.5**
**Household Composition and Survival     N = 64**
(row percentages in brackets)

|             | Survived    | Not survived | Total       |
|-------------|-------------|--------------|-------------|
| Alone       | 18 (85.7)   | 3 (14.3)     | 21 (100.0)  |
| With spouse | 31 (72.1)   | 12 (27.9)    | 43 (100.0)  |
| Total       | 49 (76.6)   | 15 (23.4)    | 64 (100.0)  |

Once more, the trend is clear, without having the further strength of statistical significance. A much higher proportion of those who lived with a spouse died than those who lived alone - more than twice as many.

Throughout the study, the importance of giving up smoking was emphasised by surgeons. Patients were being continually urged to do so, because of the contribution which smoking is believed to make to the incidence of head and neck cancer. For the purposes of the next analysis, those who have never smoked were linked with those who gave up many years ago, while those who have given up very recently were merged with those who are still smoking, since it was assumed that the clinical advantages of giving up had not yet been experienced. Table 8.6 considers the association between smoking and survival.

**Table 8.6**
**Smoking and Survival     N = 71**
(row percentages in brackets)

|            | Survived   | Not survived | Total      |
|------------|------------|--------------|------------|
| Smoker     | 29 (78.4)  | 8 (21.6)     | 37 (100.0) |
| Non Smoker | 24 (70.6)  | 10 (29.4)    | 34 (100.0) |
| Total      | 53 (74.6)  | 18 (25.4)    | 71 (100.0) |

The results were nowhere near achieving statistical significance. Remembering also that the categories had been simplified to obtain a clearer view of the trends, it can be seen that more smokers survived than non-smokers. The difference is not great, but if the results had followed the expected pattern, one would have expected a clear result in the other direction. The results may be explained in one of three ways: first, the results are not representative of the wider population; second, although smoking may contribute to morbidity, one year after onset of illness is still very early, and perhaps a different pattern might emerge after two, three or four years; third, the results may indeed be representative, and may indicate a clinical trend at variance with the accepted belief of head and neck cancer specialists.

The relationship between successful treatment (as rated by the patient) and survival was examined. It must be remembered that the views of surgeons on expected outcome and survival were not sought - this study focused on the patient perspective. What was being examined here was purely the view which the patient had about their own life chance. Table 8.7 gives the results.

**Table 8.7**
**Success of Original Treatment and Survival    N = 71**
(row percentages in brackets)

|  | Survived | Not survived | Total |
|---|---|---|---|
| Successful | 38 (76.0) | 12 (24.0) | 50 (100.0) |
| Unsuccessful | 4 (66.7) | 2 (33.3) | 6 (100.0) |
| Not Sure | 11 (73.3) | 4 (26.7) | 15 (100.0) |
| Total | 53 (74.6) | 18 (25.4) | 71 (100.0) |

The results of significance testing were very low, but nonetheless a trend is evident, namely that those who felt that treatment was successful did in fact survive to a greater extent than those who felt that treatment had not worked. Those who were not sure about outcome were similar in proportion to those who felt that treatment had succeeded.

General feeling of well-being was examined for its association with survival. Patients had been asked whether they felt better, the same, or worse than they had felt before illness. Table 8.8 gives the results.

## Table 8.8
### General Feeling of Well-being and Survival     N = 71
(row percentages in brackets)

|        | Survived    | Not survived | Total       |
|--------|-------------|--------------|-------------|
| Better | 13 (76.5)   | 4 (23.5)     | 17 (100.0)  |
| Same   | 16 (76.2)   | 5 (23.8)     | 21 (100.0)  |
| Worse  | 24 (72.7)   | 9 (27.3)     | 33 (100.0)  |
| Total  | 53 (74.6)   | 18 (25.4)    | 71 (100.0)  |

The result were virtually identical, whatever the response to the independent variable had been. Significance testing produced a very low chi squared score, but nonetheless it may be suggested that how patients felt after surgery bore little relation to whether in fact they survived. General outlook (based on the composite variable "outlook") was considered as a possible associate of survival. Table 8.9 describes the results of the analysis.

## Table 8.9
### Outlook (at First Interview) and Survival     N = 71
(row percentages in brackets)

| Outlook | Survived   | Not survived | Total      |
|---------|------------|--------------|------------|
| Low     | 8 (66.7)   | 4 (33.3)     | 12 (100.0) |
| Medium  | 28 (75.7)  | 9 (24.3)     | 37 (100.0) |
| High    | 17 (77.3)  | 5 (22.7)     | 22 (100.0) |
| Total   | 53 (74.6)  | 18 (25.4)    | 71 (100.0) |

Although no clear pattern emerged, it can be seen that those whose outlook scores had been low at the time of first interview had a somewhat higher survival rate than those whose scores had been in either the medium or high range.

The final variable considered as a possible influence on survival was satisfaction with post-operative appearance. This again was the patient's own view of their appearance. Table 8.10 gives the results.

## Table 8.10
## Satisfaction with Post-operative Appearance and Survival
## N = 71
(row percentages in brackets)

|  | Survived | Not survived | Total |
|---|---|---|---|
| Perfectly Content | 4 (76.0) | 1 (24.0) | 5 (100.0) |
| Quite Content | 20 (66.7) | 8 (33.3) | 28 (100.0) |
| Indifferent | 8 (73.3) | 4 (26.7) | 12 (100.0) |
| Dislike | 18 (66.7) | 3 (33.3) | 21 (100.0) |
| Hate | 3 (73.3) | 2 (26.7) | 5 (100.0) |
| Total | 53 (74.6) | 18 (25.4) | 71 (100.0) |

No strong pattern emerged from this analysis, which was not statistically significant. Those whose survival rates were lowest were those who had been either "quite content" or had "disliked" their post-operative appearance - that is, those who had expressed moderate views either way, rather than indifference or extreme views.

### Survival - a summary

A number of variables were considered in relation to survival. This helps describe the characteristics of those who survived, and also makes some tentative associations between survival and each of the variables - all the more tentative as none of the results reached significance:

- With the exception of those in their thirties, (all of whom survived) the older the patient, the better the survival rate;

- More women survived than men;

- A much greater proportion of white collar patients survived compared to manual workers;

225

- Those who lived in towns had twice the mortality of those who lived in the country;

- Those living with a spouse had twice the mortality rate of those who lived alone;

- More smokers survived than non-smokers;

- Those who felt that the original treatment had succeeded survived in a greater proportion than those who did not feel that it had been successful;

- How patients felt after surgery bore little relation to survival;

- Low outlook score at first interview was associated with survival;

- Those who had expressed moderate views on their post-operative appearance (either way), rather than indifference or extreme views, had the highest survival rate.

# 9 One year later

In Chapter Eight, the experience of illness and treatment was described, and the social circumstances of the 71 patients after their return home was examined. In this chapter, the focus is on the longer term: the process of recovering and rehabilitation. A year after the first interview had taken place, the treatment centres were contacted to learn whether the patients had survived. This process took place over a considerable period, since the first interviews had been staggered; patients were interviewed again a year after their first interview, rather than in one block.

The fifty-three who had survived were contacted, first by letter, and then by telephone (if this was available), to see if they would agree to a further interview. At the end of the first interview, all had said that they would be seen again, but subsequent events had deterred one from further participation.

The same format is used in this chapter as in Chapter Eight: a brief social profile of the interviewees is given, followed by details of further illness and treatment, if this has occurred. Then, their economic circumstances are described, followed by a detailed examination of their social circumstances; this includes an exploration of what has influenced their present social functioning. Next, the patients' own views on their appearance are given, together with an examination of the factors which may have influenced those views. A further section examines certain social factors in relation to fatality and survival.

In Chapter Eleven, the original hypotheses are considered, and an appraisal made of the extent to which they have been validated by empirical evidence.

## Profile of patients at time of second interview

When the second interviews were carried out, 53 of the original 71 interviewees had survived, 33 males and 20 females. This represents a survival rate of 74.6%.

Although 53 patients were still living at the time of the second interview, it must be remembered that one preferred not to be interviewed again. Consequently material derived from the follow-up interviews refers only to 52 people, 32 men and 20 women.

The ages of those who were interviewed a second time were distributed as follows:

**Table 9.1**
**Age Distribution - Second Interview    N = 52**
(column percentages in brackets)

| | | |
|---|---|---|
| 30 < 40 | 3 | (5.8) |
| 40 < 50 | 7 | (13.5) |
| 50 < 60 | 9 | (17.3) |
| 60 < 70 | 14 | (26.9) |
| 70 < 80 | 15 | (28.8) |
| 80 + | 4 | (7.7) |
| Total | 52 | (100.0) |

Table 9.2 compares the age distribution at the time of first interview and that at second interview.

**Table 9.2**
**Age Distribution - First and Second Interviews  N = 52**
(column percentages in brackets)

| | First interview | Second interview |
|---|---|---|
| 30 < 40 | 5 (7.0) | 3 (5.8) |
| 40 < 50 | 8 (11.3) | 7 (13.5) |
| 50 < 60 | 15 (21.1) | 9 (17.3) |
| 60 < 70 | 19 (26.8) | 14 (26.9) |

'continued'

| | | |
|---|---|---|
| 70 < 80 | 18 (25.4) | 15 (28.8) |
| 80+ | 6 (8.5) | 4 (7.7) |
| Total | 71 (100.0) | 52 (100.0) |

Table 9.3 describes the housing tenure of the patients at the time of the second interview.

**Table 9.3**
**Housing Tenure    N = 52**
(column percentages in brackets)

| | | |
|---|---|---|
| Owner-occupier | 14 | (26.9) |
| Own-occ.(mortgage) | 1 | (1.9) |
| Rented | 35 | (67.3) |
| Housing co-op. | 1 | (1.9) |
| Shelt. housing | 1 | (1.9) |
| Total | 52 | (100.0) |

It can be seen that virtually all the members of the sample were either owner-occupiers with no mortgage, or tenants. Few lived in any other sort of accommodation.

Seventeen of the 52, 32.6 per cent, lived alone. Of the remaining 67.3 per cent, most lived with a spouse. The proportion of those who lived alone is higher than at first interview, because of the greater number who lived with a spouse who died between first and second interview.

Seventeen surviving patients moved house between the first and second interviews. Table 9.4 describes the changes of type of area which have resulted from these moves. Due allowance must be made for slight variations in the views of interviewers of what constitutes "urban," "suburban" and "rural."

## Table 9.4
### Area of Residence - First Year's Description Compared to the Second Year    N = 52
(column and row total percentages in brackets)

First Year

| | Urban | Suburban | Rural | Total |
|---|---|---|---|---|
| Second Year | | | | |
| Urban | 9 | 1 | 1 | 11 (21.1) |
| Suburban | 11 | 16 | 6 | 33 (63.5) |
| Rural | nil | 1 | 7 | 8 (15.4) |
| Total | 20 (38.5) | 18 (34.6) | 14 (26.9) | 52 (100.0) |

The greatest fluctuations occurred in the group who at first interview were described as suburban dwellers. This could have arisen to some extent through the interviewer being uncertain how to describe the setting; even so, the re-distribution is substantial. There is no such obvious variation in those who were described first time as living in urban or rural settings.

Patients were asked whether they were happy with their standard of living - this question was aimed predominantly at the material standards within the home. The responses are summarised in Table 9.5.

## Table 9.5
### Satisfaction with Standard of Living    N = 52
(column percentages in brackets)

| | | |
|---|---|---|
| Happy | 37 | (71.1) |
| Don't mind | 11 | (21.2) |
| Not happy | 4 | (7.7) |
| Total | 52 | (100.0) |

The interviewers also expressed a view about the material standards visible within the home. Their responses are given in Table 9.6.

**Table 9.6**
**Interviewer's Rating of Living Situation  N = 52**
(column percentages in brackets)

| | | |
|---|---|---|
| Good | 29 | (55.8) |
| Sufficient | 17 | (32.7) |
| Poor | 6 | (11.5) |
| | | |
| Total | 52 | (100.0) |

It can be seen that the interviewers' ratings of material circumstances were lower than those of the patients themselves.


## Summary of profile of interviewees

At the time of the second interview, the sample was composed of 32 men and 20 women.  3.4 per cent were 60 or over. The highest mortality was found in the group in their fifties.

About a third of the patients lived alone - a slightly higher proportion than at first interview, since more died who had lived with a spouse than who lived alone.

Seventeen people had moved house since first interview. The most noticeable trend was for suburban dwellers to have moved, some into town and some to the country.

Most people were happy with their living circumstances. The interviewers' ratings of the living circumstances were slightly lower than those of the patients themselves.


## Further illness and treatment

Of the 52 patients, six reported that they had sustained a recurrence during the year. Of these, five reported that the recurrence had been treated successfully.

All of the survivors, irrespective of whether they had had a recurrence, were asked whether further treatment was anticipated. the results are given in Table 9.7.

**Table 9.7**
**Further Anticipated Treatment     N = 52**
(column percentages in brackets)

| | | |
|---|---|---|
| Yes | 6 | (11.5) |
| No | 28 | (53.8) |
| Not Sure | 18 | (34.6) |
| | | |
| Total | 52 | (100.0) |

Twenty-two reported having had a further episode in hospital during the previous year. Most of these were concerned with reconstruction. These 22 commented on whether they felt that personal help and advice was needed at a range of stages during the whole process of becoming ill and receiving treatment. The replies are given in Table 9.8.

**Table 9.8**
**When Help was Needed - The Views of Those who Received**
**Further Treatment     N = 22**
(more than one reply is possible)

| | | |
|---|---|---|
| At diagnosis | 5 | (22.7) |
| Pre-op | 4 | (18.2) |
| Post-op | 10 | (45.5) |

The 52 patients interviewed for the second time commented on their general feeling of health. This was compared to their responses shortly after surgery, at the time of the first interview. The comparison is summarised in Table 9.9.

## Table 9.9
### Since Original Illness and Treatment, Does Patient Feel Better or Worse?    N = 52
(percentage totals in brackets)

Second Year

|        | Better    | Same      | Worse     | Total First |
|--------|-----------|-----------|-----------|-------------|
| Better | 10        | 2         | 1         | 13 (25.0)   |
| Same   | 7         | 5         | 4         | 16 (30.8)   |
| Worse  | 6         | 7         | 10        | 23 (44.2)   |
| Total  | 23 (44.2) | 14 (26.9) | 15 (28.8) | 52 (100.0)  |

Many more said that they felt better after a year than they did immediately after surgery, in the previous year, 23, compared to 13. Six of those who felt worse at first interview felt better by the time of the second interview, and seven of those who felt worse subsequently reported that they then felt the same as they were before illness. Only one of those who felt better after surgery felt worse a year later.

At second interview, 17 patients (32.7%) said that they were smokers. Of those who were not, 21 (60%) had smoked in the past. Fifteen of these 21 had given up because of cancer.

At second interview, patients were asked about their alcohol consumption. Details are given in Table 9.10.

## Table 9.10
### Consumption of Alcohol    N = 52
(column percentages in brackets)

| A Lot             | 6  | (11.5)  |
|-------------------|----|---------|
| A Moderate Amount | 15 | (28.8)  |
| A Little          | 25 | (48.1)  |
| None At All       | 6  | (11.5)  |
| Total             | 52 | (100.0) |

Twenty-six of those who did drink said that they had reduced their

233

consumption since the onset of illness.

## Summary of the experience of illness and treatment

Six people reported that during the year between the interviews there had been a recurrence of cancer. Five said that this had been treated successfully.

Altogether, 22 of the patients had been in hospital during the intervening year, mostly for further reconstructive work. When these 22 were asked when help and advice were most needed, the most frequently reported time was the post- operative period. Generally, patients reported a better sense of well-being after the lapse of a year than they had done at first interview.

A third of patients were smokers. A further 21 had smoked in the past, and of these, 15 had given up since being diagnosed as having cancer. Most patients drank some alcohol, and 11.5 per cent said that they drank a lot. 26 people said that they drank less than before being ill.

## Income, work and finance

By the time of second interview, only six people were working. Of these six, the work performance of five was the same as before illness, and worse for one.

The majority of patients were not working (46 out of 52 at second interview), and were in receipt of one or more of a range of benefits. The benefits received are described in Table 9.11.

### Table 9.11
### State Benefits Received - at Second Interview    N = 46
(more than one response is possible - percentage of 46 in brackets)

| | | |
|---|---|---|
| Sickness benefit | 1 | (2.2) |
| Invalidity benefit | 18 | (39.1) |
| Attendance allowance | 4 | (8.7) |
| Mobility allowance | 1 | (2.2) |
| Income support | 3 | (6.5) |
| Retirement pension | 27 | (58.7) |

At second interview, 15 people reported a reduction in income since their original illness and treatment. Allowing for the fact that the number of interviewees was smaller than at first interview, this represents a clear increase - 28.8 per cent of interviewees compared to 18.3 per cent at first interview.

At second interview, only eight people reported that expenditure was still high. Two said that it was up to two pounds higher than before illness, five said that it was between two and five pounds more, and one said that it was eighteen pounds higher.

### Summary of economic issues

Only six people were working by the time of the second interviews. One, a man, said that his performance at work had deteriorated.

The remainder all received state benefits; more than half received retirement pension, and over a third received invalidity benefit.

Income had reduced for 28.8 per cent. This represents deterioration both since illness and since the first interview. Fewer people reported raised expenditure.

### Social and personal functioning

Thirty-six of the 52 survivors, 69.2 per cent, pursued social and leisure activities outside the house. However, 27, 51.9 per cent were now more restricted in the leisure activities which they felt able to pursue, as a result of illness and treatment.

In other ways, however, for example within the home, matters were somewhat more positive. Table 9.12 describes the patients' rating of their ability to carry out home responsibilities.

### Table 9.12
### Carrying out Home Responsibilities - a Year On   N = 52
(column percentages in brackets)

| | | |
|---|---|---|
| Better | 2 | (3.8) |
| Same | 34 | (65.3) |
| Worse | 16 | (30.8) |

It can be seen that there had been a functional improvement for some - at second interview only 30.0 per cent were functioning at a lower level than before illness, compared to 47.9 per cent at first interview.

Table 9.13 considers the relationship with the patient's spouse. The question of change was asked in relation to the situation at time of interview compared to before illness and surgery.

### Table 9.13
### Relations with Spouse - a Year On    N = 28
(column percentages in brackets)

| | | |
|---|---|---|
| Better | 11 | (39.3) |
| The same | 14 | (50.0) |
| Worse | 3 | (10.7) |
| | | |
| Total | 28 | (100.0) |

It can be seen that few felt that relations had deteriorated. If anything, the experience had had an enhancing effect on a substantial number of the sample.

The third of the social functioning factors, use of community resources, was again asked in comparison to the situation before the original illness and surgery. Table 9.14 gives the results.

### Table 9.14
### Use of Community Resources - a Year On    N = 52
(column percentages in brackets)

| | | |
|---|---|---|
| More | 4 | (7.7) |
| The same | 33 | (63.4) |
| Less | 15 | (28.8) |
| | | |
| Total | 52 | (100.0) |

For most, there had been no change in the extent to which they had used community resources. However, for 28.8 per cent there had been a deterioration.

The three areas of functioning described in the previous three tables were the same as those used to compute the variable "Social Functioning" in the first year analysis. The same computation was carried out, and a number of variables cross-tabulated with the new variable, in order to see whether they had any influence on social functioning.

The new social functioning scale had a potential score ranging from three to fifteen. In fact all the scores fell between three and ten. In the following scale the scores have been simplified in order to see trends more clearly. Scores up to six are described as "low", and scores of seven and over are described as "high".

Table 9.15 considers the relationship between age and social functioning. Percentages have not been calculated, because of the low numbers involved in each cell.

### Table 9.15
### Age and Social Functioning   N = 52

Social Functioning

| Age | Low | High |
|---|---|---|
| 30 < 40 | 2 | 1 |
| 40 < 50 | 2 | |
| 50 < 60 | 3 | 6 |
| 60 < 70 | 4 | 10 |
| 70 < 80 | 8 | 7 |
| 80 + | 1 | 3 |
| Total | 52 | (100.0) |

The results were significant - chi-squared = 44.01 at a probability level of .04756. The younger patients, aged below 50, tended to function more poorly than those aged 50 to 70. Thereafter there is again a lowering of standard of functioning. However, this could to some extent be associated with a general influence of age on functional ability.

The influence of gender on social functioning was then considered. Table 9.16 describes the results.

**Table 9.16**
**Gender and Social Functioning    N = 52**
(row percentages in brackets)

Social Functioning

|        | Low        | High       | Total |
|--------|------------|------------|-------|
| Male   | 16 (50.0)  | 16 (50.0)  | 32    |
| Female | 7 (35.0)   | 13 (65.0)  | 20    |
| Total  | 23 (44.2)  | 29 (55.8)  | 52    |

The results were not statistically significant. However, more women were functioning at a higher level than men, who were divided evenly between low functioning and high.

The question of isolation was then addressed. Those living alone were compared to those who lived with someone, particularly with spouses, and related to social functioning. The results, which were almost significant (chi squared = 20.2 at probability level of .06409), are given in Table 9.17.

**Table 9.17**
**Isolation and Social Functioning    N = 52**
(row percentages in brackets)

Social Functioning

|                   | Low        | High       | Total |
|-------------------|------------|------------|-------|
| Lives Alone       | 4 (23.5)   | 13 (76.5)  | 17    |
| Lives With Others | 19 (54.3)  | 16 (45.7)  | 35    |
| Total             | 23 (44.2)  | 29 (55.8)  | 52    |

There is a strong difference in the social functioning of those who live alone compared to those who live with others. Those who live alone were functioning at a substantially higher level. This is particularly remarkable since those who lived alone were not able to contribute a score to one of the components of the social functioning scale, namely relations with spouse.

Social class was then considered as a possible influence on social functioning. Table 9.18 summarises the findings. The social class variable has been condensed into the two values "white collar" and "manual."

## Table 9.18
### Social Class and Social Functioning   N = 52
(row percentages in brackets)

Social Functioning

|  | Low | High | Total |
|---|---|---|---|
| White Collar | 5 (33.3) | 10 (66.7) | 15 |
| Manual | 18 (48.6) | 19 (51.3) | 37 |
| Total | 23 (44.2) | 29 (55.8) | 52 |

The results were not significant. Those of higher social class functioned somewhat better than those of manual occupations.

Patients had been asked how they felt in general terms at the time of interview. This was considered as a possible influence on social functioning. The analysis is summarised in Table 9.19.

## Table 9.19
### Well-being and Social Functioning   N = 52
(row percentages in brackets)

Social Functioning

|  | Low | High | Total |
|---|---|---|---|
| Better | 13 (56.5) | 10 (43.5) | 23 |
| Same | 7 (50.0) | 7 (50.0) | 14 |
| Worse | 3 (20.0) | 12 (80.0) | 15 |
| Total | 23 (44.2) | 29 (55.8) | 52 |

Those who said that they felt better than before were functioning at a lower level than those who were feeling worse. The latter were functioning at a level substantially higher than any other group. However, the results did not achieve significance, and so must be treated with caution.

The issue of outlook was then considered, in relation to social functioning a year after treatment. First of all, outlook at the time of first interview was examined. It will be remembered that the variable "Outlook" was composed of three variables, which were merged to provide a more robust indicator of mood and attitude. Table 9.20 summarises the responses.

**Table 9.20**
**Outlook at First Interview and Social Functioning    N = 52**
(row percentages in brackets)

Social Functioning

| Outlook | Low | High | Total |
|---|---|---|---|
| Low | 2 (25.0) | 6 (75.0) | 8 |
| Medium | 10 (37.0) | 17 (63.0) | 27 |
| High | 11 (64.7) | 6 (35.3) | 17 |
| Total | 23 (44.2) | 29 (55.8) | 52 |

It can be seen that there is a fairly strong inverse association between outlook at time of first interview and social functioning at time of second interview. The results were near to significance -chi squared = 4.6 at a probability level of .09754.

Outlook a year later was then considered, to see whether current outlook correlated with social functioning as described at the same interview. The results are given in Table 9.21.

### Table 9.21
### Outlook at Second Interview and Social Functioning $\quad$ N = 52
(row percentages in brackets)

Social Functioning

| Outlook | Low | High | Total |
|---|---|---|---|
| Low | nil | 3 (100.0) | 3 |
| Medium | 2 (14.3) | 12 (85.7) | 14 |
| High | 21 (60.0) | 14 (40.0) | 35 |
| Total | 23 (44.2) | 29 (55.8) | 52 |

The results were highly significant - chi squared = 10.9 at a probability level of .00409. There was a strong inverse association between outlook at second interview and social functioning at second interview. Those whose outlook was positive functioned at a lower level than the rest.

The influence of change in outlook between the two interviews on social functioning was not so clear, and the results of this analysis did not achieve significance.

Patients had been asked whether people had changed in their attitude to them since surgery, and this was now considered as a possible influence on social functioning. Table 9.22 gives the results.

### Table 9.22
### Change in the Attitude of Others and Social Functioning
### N = 52
(row percentages in brackets)

Social Functioning

| Attitude Changed? | Low | High | Total |
|---|---|---|---|
| Changed | 11 (36.7) | 19 (63.3) | 30 |
| Unchanged | 12 (54.5) | 10 (45.5) | 22 |
| Total | 23 (44.2) | 29 (55.8) | 52 |

The results were not significant. Those who said that people had changed in their attitude to them also reported a somewhat higher level of social functioning.

The previous tables described the relationship of certain important variables to social functioning at the time of second interview. In addition, since the questions which formed the social functioning scale were asked at first and second interviews, it was possible to compute the difference between felt level of social functioning at first interview and that experienced at second. The same variables were then applied, to see whether they influenced change in functioning.

First, the effect of age was considered. This analysis produced little of interest: the results did not achieve a high statistical significance (chi squared = 42.7 at a probability level of .17358). Those whose functioning had reduced were fairly balanced by those for whom it had improved, and largely, this was balanced at all age levels. Age did not seem to have a major impact in change in functioning.

Next, gender was considered, and its possible impact on social functioning. The results are described in Table 9.23.

**Table 9.23**
**Gender and Change in Social Functioning    N = 52**
(row percentages in brackets)

Social Functioning

|  | Lower | The Same | Higher |
|---|---|---|---|
| Male | 14 (43.8) | 9 (28.1) | 9 (28.1) |
| Female | 6 (30.0) | 4 (20.0) | 10 (50.0) |
| Total | 20 (38.5) | 13 (25.0) | 19 (36.5) |

The results were significant (chi-squared = 14.7 at a probability level of .04035). Half of the women had improved their social functioning score, compared to not much more than a quarter of men. Forty-three per cent of men had deteriorated, while only 30 per cent of women had done so. It can be seen therefore, with the added conviction of statistical significance, that the social functioning of women was considerably more positive in direction than that of men.

The living situation of the patients was then considered. Those who

242

lived alone were compared to those who lived with others. Table 9.24 gives the results.

## Table 9.24
### Living Situation and Change in Social Functioning  N = 52
(row percentages in brackets)

Social Functioning

|  | Lower | The Same | Higher |
|---|---|---|---|
| Alone | 3 (17.6) | 4 (23.5) | 10 (58.8) |
| Not Alone | 17 (48.6) | 9 (25.7) | 9 (25.7) |
| Total | 20 (38.5) | 13 (25.0) | 19 (36.5) |

The results were verging on significance (chi squared = 20.9 at a probability level of .10424). Around a quarter of the patients, whether living alone or with someone else, had not varied their social functioning either for better or worse. However, many of those who lived alone (more than half) had improved their score, contrasted with a quarter of those who lived with someone else. Almost half (48.6 per cent) of those who lived with someone had deteriorated, compared to 17.6 per cent of those who lived alone.

In considering the effect of social class on changed social functioning, as on previous occasions, the social class categories were simplified to "white collar" and "manual". The results are given in Table 9.25.

## Table 9.25
### Social Class and Change in Social Functioning    N = 52
(row percentages in brackets)

Social Functioning

|  | Lower | The Same | Higher |
|---|---|---|---|
| White Collar | 5 (33.3) | 2 (13.3) | 8 (53.3) |
| Manual | 15 (40.5) | 11 (29.7) | 11 (29.7) |
| Total | 20 (38.5) | 13 (25.0) | 19 (36.5) |

The results of this analysis were not significant. Taking this into account, it can be said tentatively that white collar patients had improved their functioning more than manual patients. More of the latter had either stayed the same or deteriorated than the white collar group.

Next, the question of whether patients felt better or worse than before illness and treatment was examined for its effect on changed social functioning. The results were not significant, and no clear pattern was evident.

Once more, outlook was considered, and this in three stages, as before. First, the effect of outlook at first interview was considered on the extent of change in social functioning between the two interviews. Table 9.26 gives the results.

## Table 9.26
### Outlook (at First Interview) and Change in Social Functioning
### N = 52
(row percentages in brackets)

Social Functioning

|  | Lower | The Same | Higher |
|---|---|---|---|
| Outlook |  |  |  |
| Low | 5 (62.5) | nil | 3 (37.5) |

'continued'

| | | | |
|---|---|---|---|
| Medium | 7 (25.9) | 10 (37.0) | 10 (37.0) |
| High | 8 (47.1) | 3 (17.6) | 6 (35.3) |
| | | | |
| Total | 20 (38.5) | 13 (25.0) | 19 (36.5) |

The results were verging on significance - chi squared = 6.5 at a probability level of .16011. Although the trend was not straightforward, there was some suggestion that those whose outlook scores were low at first interview had deteriorated in their functioning more than those whose outlook score had been high. Those whose functioning score had deteriorated least were those whose outlook at first interview had been moderate.

The same analysis was carried out for the outlook scale derived from second interviews, and their effect on changed social functioning. The results are given in Table 9.27.

**Table 9.27**
**Outlook (at Second Interview) and Change in Social Functioning**
**N = 52**
(row percentages in brackets)

| Social Functioning | Lower | The Same | Higher |
|---|---|---|---|
| Outlook | | | |
| Low | 1 (33.3) | nil | 1 (66.7) |
| Medium | 5 (35.7) | 3 (21.4) | 6 (42.9) |
| High | 14 (40.0) | 10 (28.6) | 11 (31.4) |
| | | | |
| Total | 20 (38.5) | 13 (25.0) | 19 (36.5) |

This analysis did not achieve statistical significance. Again, no absolute trend could be seen, but there was a slight tendency towards an inverse relationship between outlook at second interview and changed social functioning; as outlook improved, social functioning changed for the worse.

Finally in this consideration of the effect of outlook on changed social functioning, the effect of changed outlook was considered for its influence on functioning. This is described in Table 9.28.

## Table 9.28
### Change in Outlook and Change in Social Functioning    N = 52
(row percentages in brackets)

Social Functioning

| Outlook | Lower | The Same | Higher |
|---|---|---|---|
| Lower | 2 (28.6) | nil | 5 (71.4) |
| Same | 4 (50.0) | 1 (12.5) | 3 (37.5) |
| Higher | 14 (37.8) | 12 (32.4) | 11 (29.7) |
| Total | 20 (38.5) | 13 (25.0) | 19 (36.5) |

The results were approaching significance - chi squared = 6.3 at a probability level of .17538. As with the absolute scores for outlook at second interview, so with the change in outlook - there was something of a tendency for deteriorated outlook to be associated with improved social functioning; again too there was some slight inverse association between improved outlook and improved social functioning.

The final analysis in the section on social functioning considered the effect of the attitude of others on the extent of changed social functioning of the patients. The results were not remarkable: they were not statistically significant, and there was little clear trend.

## Outlook

It will be remembered that at first interview stage, a series of three questions addressed the issue of mood and outlook. Similar questions were asked at second interview. The same question about sense of fulfilment was asked. Next, patients were asked about their attitude to the future. This was intended as a slightly refined version of the previous year's question about optimism. The third question, about day-to-day mood, was intended to correspond broadly to the question of the previous year about enthusiasm for life. First of all, day-to-day mood was considered. Responses to each question were placed on a five-point scale (by the respondents themselves), five being the most positive outlook, and one being the lowest possible. When recording responses to the day-to-day mood question, allowance was also made for the fact that for many it is normal to have a fluctuating mood pattern. Day-to-day mood was examined first, and Table 9.29 describes the responses.

**Table 9.29**
**Day-to-day Mood    N = 52**
(column percentages in brackets)

| Positive | 12 | (23.1) |
|---|---|---|
| 4 | 12 | (23.1) |
| 3 | 7 | (13.5) |
| 2 | 4 | (7.7) |
| Negative | 4 | (7.7) |
| Up & Down | 13 | (25.0) |

It can be seen that as a general pattern, mood was described as positive. Twenty-five per cent took the opportunity provided to record that their mood swung up and down.

The question about sense of fulfilment in life was repeated in exactly the form used in the first interview. The replies are given in Table 9.30.

**Table 9.30**
**Sense of Fulfilment    N = 52**
(column percentages in brackets)

| Positive | 18 | (34.6) |
|---|---|---|
| 4 | 13 | (25.0) |
| 3 | 12 | (23.1) |
| 2 | 8 | (15.4) |
| Negative | 1 | (1.9) |

Once more, the overall response was positive - more than half the responses were recorded on either point four or point five.

The patients were then asked what their attitude was to the future. As suggested above, this was intended as a slightly refined version of the previous year's question about level of optimism. The responses are given in Table 9.31.

**Table 9.31**
**Attitude to the Future    N = 52**
(column percentages in brackets)

| Positive | 14 | (26.9) |
|----------|----|--------|
| 4        | 14 | (26.9) |
| 3        | 15 | (28.8) |
| 2        | 6  | (11.5) |
| Negative | 3  | (5.8)  |

A very similar proportion gave a positive response. Without ignoring those who scored low in their responses, it can be seen that the overall picture is not one of bleakness about the future - rather one of equanimity or even better.

It will be remembered that in presentation of the results of the first year interviews, the three variables relating to outlook were merged to form one composite variable known as "outlook". The same variable was computed for the second year findings. Once more, a 15-point scale was obtained, with a possible range of scores from three to 15. In fact, a range from three to 13 was scored. The mean score was 8.0. In presentation of the results, the scores have been summarised into the categories "low", "medium" and "high".

First, the influence on age on outlook at time of second interview was considered. The results are summarised in Table 9.32 Percentages are not calculated because of the small numbers in most cells.

**Table 9.32**
**Age and Outlook (Second Interview)    N = 52**
(row percentages in brackets)

Outlook

| Age | Low | Medium | High |
|-----|-----|--------|------|
| 30 < 40 | nil | 1 | 2 |

248

'continued'

| | | | |
|---|---|---|---|
| 40 < 50 | 1 | 1 | 5 |
| 50 < 60 | 1 | 3 | 5 |
| 60 < 70 | 1 | 5 | 8 |
| 70 < 80 | nil | 3 | 12 |
| 80+ | nil | 1 | 3 |

The results were not significant, and little pattern was evident, from which it may be assumed that age affected outlook very little, at the time of second interview.

Next, the influence of gender on outlook was examined. Table 9.33 describes the findings.

**Table 9.33**
**Gender and Outlook (Second Interview)    N = 52**
(row percentages in brackets)

Outlook

| | Low | Medium | High |
|---|---|---|---|
| Male | 1  (3.1) | 10 (31.3) | 21 (65.6) |
| Female | 2 (10.0) | 4 (20.0) | 14 (70.0) |
| Total | 3  (5.8) | 14 (26.9) | 35 (67.3) |

The results did not reach significance, and there was little evidence of either men or women being more positive in outlook than each other.

The issue of isolation was then considered, by investigating the effect on outlook of living alone or living with others. This investigation is reviewed in Table 9.34.

## Table 9.34
## Living Situation and Outlook (Second Interview)
## N = 52
(row percentages in brackets)

Outlook

|  | Low | Medium | High |
|---|---|---|---|
| Alone | 2 (11.8) | 4 (23.5) | 11 (64.7) |
| With Others | 1 (2.9) | 10 (28.6) | 24 (68.6) |
| Total | 3 (5.8) | 14 (26.9) | 35 (67.3) |

The results were verging on significance; chi squared = 7.9 at a probability level of .09195. There was evidence of a slight trend towards the outlook scores of those who lived with others being higher than those who lived alone.

The effect of social class on outlook was considered. As on previous occasions, social class categories have been simplified into two values, white collar and manual. Table 9.35 summarises the findings.

## Table 9.35
## Social Class and Outlook (Second Interview)
## N = 52
(row percentages in brackets)

Outlook

|  | Low | Medium | High |
|---|---|---|---|
| White Collar | 1 (6.7) | 3 (20.0) | 11 (73.3) |
| Manual | 2 (5.4) | 11 (29.7) | 24 (64.9) |
| Total | 3 (5.8) | 14 (26.9) | 35 (67.3) |

The results were not statistically significant. White collar workers reported somewhat higher scores than manual workers on outlook.

Area of residence was considered as a possible influence on outlook. Table 9.36 describes the results of the analysis.

## Table 9.36
## Area and Outlook (Second Interview)    N = 52
### (row percentages in brackets)

Outlook

|          | Low        | Medium     | High        |
|----------|------------|------------|-------------|
| Urban    | 3 (15.0)   | 5 (25.0)   | 12 (60.0)   |
| Suburban | nil        | 6 (33.3)   | 12 (66.7)   |
| Rural    | nil        | 3 (21.4)   | 11 (78.6)   |
| Total    | 3  (5.8)   | 14 (26.9)  | 35 (67.3)   |

The results were not significant, but a distinct trend is evident whereby outlook is substantially lower for those who live in towns, especially contrasted with country-dwellers. The low scores in the rural category make the results somewhat unreliable.

Other environmental issues were considered at second interview, and these were now examined as possible influences on outlook. The first was type of accommodation (house, flat or bungalow).

The results were not significant, and they did not describe any strong trend.

Next, housing tenure was considered, and its association with outlook. Table 9.37 summarises the results.

## Table 9.37
## Tenure and Outlook (Second Interview)
## N = 52
### (row percentages in brackets)

Outlook

|          | Low       | Medium    | High       |
|----------|-----------|-----------|------------|
| Own-occ. | 1 (7.1)   | 4 (28.6)  | 9 (64.3)   |
| Mortgage | nil       | nil       | 1          |
| Rented   | 1 (2.9)   | 9 (25.7)  | 25 (71.4)  |
| Co-op.   | nil       | 1         | nil        |
| Other    | 1         | nil       | nil        |
| Total    | 3 (5.8)   | 14 (26.9) | 35 (67.3)  |

Percentages were only calculated for owner occupier and rented accommodation. Other tenure type scores were negligible. The results were highly significant - chi squared = 20.2 at a probability level of .00949. They suggested that those living in rented property had a more positive outlook than those who owned their own house.

Most people were content with their material conditions - their house and furnishings; 71 per cent said that they were happy, and 21 per cent said that they didn't mind; only 8 per cent were not happy with their living conditions. These responses were analysed in relation to outlook at time of second interview, and some highly significant results were produced - chi squared = 25.6 at a probability level of .00004. Table 9.38 gives the results.

**Table 9.38**
**Satisfaction with Living Situation and Outlook**
**(Second Interview)    N = 52**
(row percentages in brackets)

Outlook

| | Low | Medium | High |
|---|---|---|---|
| Happy | 1 (2.7) | 6 (16.2) | 30 (81.1) |
| Don't Mind | nil | 7 (63.6) | 4 (36.4) |
| Not Happy | 2 (50.0) | 1 (25.0) | 1 (25.0) |
| Total | 3 (5.8) | 14 (26.9) | 35 (67.3) |

There was a strong and very clear association between the patient's contentment with their living situation and their overall outlook on life. Interviewers were also asked to give their view of material standards in the home. Their ratings were slightly lower - 56 per cent were described as having good material standards, 33 per cent sufficient, and 11 per cent poor standards. These findings too were matched with outlook scores, and again, the results were highly significant - chi squared = 13.5 at a probability level of .00892. Table 9.39 gives the results.

## Table 9.39
### Interviewer Opinion of Living Situation and Outlook
### (Second Interview)    N = 52
(row percentages in brackets)

Outlook

|            | Low      | Medium     | High      |
|------------|----------|------------|-----------|
| Good       | 2 (6.9)  | 3 (10.3)   | 24 (82.8) |
| Sufficient | nil      | 7 (41.2)   | 10 (58.8) |
| Poor       | 1 (16.7) | 4 (66.7)   | 1 (16.7)  |
| Total      | 3 (5.8)  | 14 (26.9)  | 35 (67.3) |

Again, there was a strong positive association between the living situation (this time rated by the interviewer) and the patient's outlook on life.

Patients had been asked how they felt generally at second interview, compared to before illness. The association between their responses to this question and overall outlook was next examined. The results are summarised in Table 9.40.

## Table 9.40
### Well-being and Outlook (Second Interview)
### N = 52
(row percentages in brackets)

Outlook

|        | Low      | Medium     | High      |
|--------|----------|------------|-----------|
| Better | nil      | 5 (21.7)   | 18 (78.3) |
| Same   | nil      | 2 (14.3)   | 12 (85.7) |
| Worse  | 3 (20.0) | 7 (46.7)   | 5 (33.3)  |
| Total  | 3 (5.8)  | 14 (26.9)  | 35 (67.3) |

The results were highly significant - chi squared = 14.3 at a probability level of .00634. Those who felt better also had a very positive outlook, but not to the extent of those who felt the same as before - perhaps the message is that equanimity is more useful than a substantial improvement in mood. Those who felt worse than before tended to have moderate outlook scores.

Whether an individual felt better was not necessarily related to actual illness. The patients were therefore asked directly whether they understood a recurrence to have occurred. Table 9.41 gives the results.

**Table 9.41**
**Recurrence of Illness and Outlook (Second Interview)    N = 52**
(row percentages in brackets)

Outlook

|  | Low | Medium | High |
| --- | --- | --- | --- |
| Further Illness | 1 (16.7) | 3 (50.0) | 2 (33.3) |
| None | 2 (4.3) | 11 (23.9) | 33 (71.7) |
| Total | 3 (5.8) | 14 (26.9) | 35 (67.3) |

The results were approaching significance - chi squared = 3.9 at a probability level of .14221. Those for whom there had been a recurrence were small in number, but it can be said that they were more likely to have a low outlook score.

Patients had been asked whether they felt that their appearance had changed since first illness and surgery. Their responses were examined for a possible association with outlook.  The results were not significant, but there was nevertheless some suggestion that those who felt that their appearance had changed were not so positive in their outlook as those who felt that surgery had changed their appearance.

**Change in outlook between first and second interview**

The same group of variables whose relationship with outlook at the time of second interview has just been described were further considered in relation to the change which might have occurred in the patients' outlook between first and second interview. The changed outlook score was obtained by subtracting the score for outlook at second interview from the score at first interview. For a little more than half of the surviving patients, 54 per cent, outlook scores had deteriorated. In the following tables, the outlook difference is summarised as "worse", "the same" or "better". The variables are considered in exactly the same order as in the previous section. Only those analyses which produced clear patterns or statistical significance are described in detail.

First, the effect of age on changed outlook was considered. The results were not significant, but they suggest that between the two interviews, outlook had generally changed for the better, and this was strikingly so in the instance of those in their seventies (93.3 per cent in this age group had improved their outlook score).

Next, the influence of gender on changed outlook was examined. The results were not significant. Nor was any strong difference evident between men and women.

The issue of isolation was then considered, by investigating the effect of living alone or living with others on outlook. This investigation is reported in Table 9.42.

### Table 9.42
### Living Situation and Changed Outlook     N = 52
(row percentages in brackets)

| Outlook | Worse | Same | Higher |
|---|---|---|---|
| Alone | 5 (29.4) | 2 (11.8) | 10 (58.8) |
| With Others | 2 (5.7) | 6 (17.6) | 27 (77.1) |
| Total | 7 (13.5) | 8 (15.4) | 37 (31.2) |

The results were highly significant; chi squared = 15.2 at a probability level of .00426. They suggested that those who lived with others were far more likely to have changed their outlook scores for the better than those who lived alone. Although more than half of those who lived alone had improved their outlook scores, there was still a large proportion (29 per cent) whose outlook was less positive than at first interview.

The effect of social class on outlook was considered. This is described in Table 9.43.

Table 9.43
## Social Class and Changed Outlook    N = 52
(row percentages in brackets)

Outlook

|  | Worse | Same | Better |
|---|---|---|---|
| White Collar | 3 (20.0) | 3 (20.0) | 9 (60.0) |
| Manual | 4 (10.8) | 5 (13.5) | 28 (75.7) |
| Total | 7 (13.5) | 8 (15.4) | 37 (31.2) |

The results were not significant. However, a strong difference can be seen between the two groups; a far smaller proportion of white collar workers had improved their outlook scores compared to manual workers.

Area of residence was next considered as a possible influence on changed outlook. The results were not significant, but there was something of a trend evident that rural dwellers were most likely to have deteriorated outlook scores, and the most positive were urban dwellers.

Type of accommodation (house, flat or bungalow) was then examined as a possible influence on outlook. As in the previous analysis of this variable, the results were not significant, and the slight trend evident must be treated with caution, namely the tendency for those who lived in bungalows to have reduced their outlook scores more than others. The changes for the better were virtually the same for those in houses and in flats.

Next, the association of housing tenure was considered. Table 9.44 summarises the results.

## Table 9.44
## Tenure and Changed Outlook    N = 52
(row percentages in brackets)

Outlook

|  | Worse | Same | Better |
|---|---|---|---|
| Own-occ. | 4 (28.6) | 3 (21.4) | 7 (50.0) |

'continued'

| | | | |
|---|---|---|---|
| Mortgage | nil | nil | 1 |
| Rented | 3 (8.6) | 4 (11.4) | 28 (80.0) |
| Co-op. | nil | nil | 1 |
| Other | nil | 1 | nil |
| Total | 7 (13.5) | 8 (15.4) | 37 (31.2) |

Percentages were only calculated for owner occupier and rented accommodation. Other tenure type scores were negligible. The results were approaching significance - chi squared $= 11.3$ at a probability level of .18735. It will be remembered that there was a very high level of significance reported in the association between tenure and outlook at second interview. This is borne out in this analysis of changed outlook. Those in rented property improved their outlook scores between the two interviews dramatically more than those who were owner-occupiers.

The association between patient satisfaction with their living situation and change in outlook was examined. The results are given in Table 9.45.

**Table 9.45**
**Satisfaction with Living Situation and Changed Outlook  N = 52**
(row percentages in brackets)

Outlook

| | Worse | Same | Better |
|---|---|---|---|
| Happy | 6 (16.2) | 4 (10.8) | 27 (73.0) |
| Don't Mind | nil | 2 (18.2) | 9 (81.8) |
| Not Happy | 1 (25.0) | 2 (50.0) | 1 (25.0) |
| Total | 7 (13.5) | 8 (15.4) | 37 (31.2) |

The results were approaching significance - chi squared $= 7.1$ at a probability level of .12817. Most people were happy with their living situation (71 per cent) and therefore the results for those who did not mind it or who were happy must be interpreted cautiously. However, they seem to suggest that those who were not happy with their material surroundings tended to have stayed the same in their outlook between the two interviews. Those who did not mind changed for the better in most instances, as did those who were happy with their circumstances.

Interviewers were asked to give their own view of living standards in the home. Their responses, which scored lower than those of the patients themselves, were matched with changed outlook scores. The results, which did not reach significance, are given in Table 9.46.

## Table 9.46
## Interviewer Opinion of Living Situation and Changed Outlook
## N = 52
(row percentages in brackets)

Outlook

|  | Worse | Same | Better |
|---|---|---|---|
| Good | 4 (13.8) | 4 (13.8) | 21 (72.4) |
| Sufficient | 2 (11.8) | 4 (23.5) | 11 (64.7) |
| Poor | 1 (16.7) | nil | 5 (83.3) |
| Total | 7 (13.5) | 8 (15.4) | 37 (31.2) |

The pattern was not distinctive, but it can be seen that those whose circumstances were described by the interviewer as "sufficient" were the most likely to have deteriorated outlook scores. Those whose scores were most likely to have increased were those whose circumstances were described as "poor".

The relationship between general feeling of well-being and change in outlook was next considered. No clear trend was evident; nor were the results significant. Those who felt the same as before illness seemed to have fared best, while those who felt either better or worse described similar outlook changes to each other.

Patients were then asked directly whether they understood a recurrence to have occurred. Table 9.47 gives the results of an analysis of the results of this question in relation to changed outlook scores.

## Table 9.47
### Recurrence of Illness and Changed Outlook　　N = 52
(row percentages in brackets)

Outlook

|  | Low | Medium | High |
| --- | --- | --- | --- |
| Further Illness | 1 (16.7) | 1 (16.7) | 4 (66.7) |
| None | 6 (13.0) | 7 (15.2) | 33 (71.7) |
| Total | 7 (13.5) | 8 (15.4) | 37 (31.2) |

The results were not significant, and the numbers who reported further illness were low, so it is difficult to rely on the analysis. As it stands, there was little difference in reported change in outlook between those who had sustained a recurrence and those who had been free from further episodes.

Patients' views on whether they felt that their appearance had changed since first illness and surgery were examined for a possible association with outlook. Table 9.48 gives the results.

## Table 9.48
### Changed Appearance and Changed Outlook
### N = 52
(row percentages in brackets)

Outlook

|  | Worse | Same | Better |
| --- | --- | --- | --- |
| Changed | 7 (17.9) | 6 (15.4) | 26 (66.7) |
| Unchanged | nil | 2 (15.4) | 11 (84.6) |
| Total | 7 (13.5) | 8 (15.4) | 37 (31.2) |

The results did not achieve significance. Chi squared = 2.8 at a probability level of .24973. However, it can be seen that those who felt that their appearance had changed tended to have improved their

259

outlook scores far less than those who felt that there had been no change.

## Summary of social consequences

More than half of the sample were more restricted than previously in their leisure activities. The proportion of those who could fulfil responsibilities within the house had improved.

Several people felt that relations with their spouse had improved.

There was considerable deterioration (28.8 per cent) in use of community resources.

When social functioning at second interview was examined more closely, a series of variables was examined for their impact or influence on it. The following is a summary of this analysis:

- Those aged up to 50 functioned more poorly than those aged 50 to 70;

- Women tended to function at a higher level than men;

- Many of those who lived alone functioned at a higher level than those who lived with others;

- White collar workers functioned better than manual workers;

- That those who felt better in themselves actually functioned worse in practical terms;

- Outlook seemed inversely related to social functioning. Positive outlook at first and second interviews was associated with poor functioning scores;

- The patients who felt that others had changed their attitude to them for the worse tended to report a high level of functioning.

When change in social functioning between the two interviews was considered, the same group of variables was considered a second time, to see what if any impact they had on, or what association they had with, this change. The analysis produced the following results:

- Age had little effect on change in functioning;

- Women had improved their functioning scores substantially more than men (the analysis was statistically significant);

- Those who lived alone had improved their social functioning more than those who lived with someone else;

- Patients with "white collar" backgrounds had improved their functioning more than patients with manual backgrounds;

- A general feeling of well-being seemed to have little association with change in social functioning;

- There was some indication that those who scored low on outlook at first interview had poorer social functioning than those whose outlook scores had been high, while those with better outlook scores seemed to have changed their social functioning scores for the worse.

Outlook itself was a variable composed of three variables related to psychological functioning: generally, day-to-day mood was described as positive, and the responses to the other two "outlook" variables, namely fulfilment and attitude to the future, also tended towards the positive end of the scale. The following is a summary of the analysis of a range of variables in relation to the composite outlook variable:

- Age and gender had little effect on outlook at second interview;

- The outlook scores of those living alone were slightly higher than of those who lived with someone else;

- White collar workers reported slightly higher outlook scores than manual workers;

- The outlook scores of those who lived in towns was much lower than of other groups. The type of house in which the person lived seemed not to have any influence, but those who lived in rented property had a significantly better outlook than owner-occupiers;

- If people were content with their living situation, they tended to display a positive outlook. Similarly, if the interviewer reported good material circumstances, this too was associated with a high outlook score;

- Sense of well-being was significantly associated with high outlook score, but the most positive were those who felt the same as before, rather than those who felt better. In addition, those for whom there had been a further occurrence of cancer tended to report a poorer outlook;

- A feeling that appearance had changed for the worse was also associated with poor outlook.

Between the two interviews, generally, outlook had changed for the better. The next series of conclusions refers to the extent to which the variables in question were associated with a change in outlook between the first and second interviews:

- This improvement was particularly noticeable for those in their seventies;

- There was little sign of gender difference in changed outlook scores;

- Those who lived with others were far more likely to have improved their outlook scores than those who lived alone;

- A smaller proportion of white collar workers had improved their outlook than manual workers;

- Country dwellers were most likely to have poorer outlook scores; urban dwellers showed the most positive changes;

- Those living in rented property had improved their

outlook far more than had owner-occupiers;

- Satisfaction with living situation tended to be associated positively with outlook change; however, interviewer rating of living circumstances was inversely related to changed outlook;

- Sense of well-being (compared to the situation before illness) was not directly associated with improved outlook;

- A recurrence of cancer seemed not to cause outlook to change either for better or worse;

- Those who felt that their appearance had changed through illness and surgery had reduced their outlook scores.


**Appearance**

As at the first interview, patients were asked for their views on their own appearance. They were asked how they had felt about their appearance before the original surgery, and how they felt about their appearance now. On both occasions, they were asked to rate their appearance on a five-point scale, as follows:

- Perfectly content;
- Quite content;
- Indifferent;
- Dislike;
- Hate.

Table 9.49 shows in graph form the contrast between ratings at first interview and ratings at second. First interview ratings are on the left of the pair, second on the right. Please see following page.

# Table 9.49
## Satisfaction with Appearance - Past and Present    N = 52

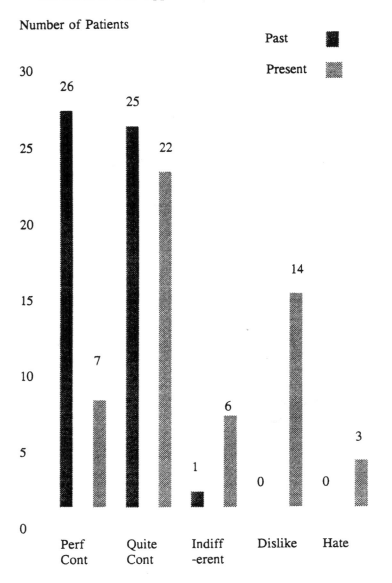

Number of Patients

Past ■

Present ▨

It can be seen that most people had been either perfectly content or quite content with their previous appearance, while there many at second interview (14) who actively disliked it. More were indifferent at second interview than at first.

Table 9.50 explores the change further by describing how much difference was experienced between the point before surgery and the time of second interview.

**Table 9.50**
**Felt Difference Between Before Surgery and Time of Second Interview   N = 52**
(column percentages in brackets)

| | | |
|---|---|---|
| 1 point up | 1 | (1.9) |
| no different | 20 | (38.5) |
| 1 point down | 11 | (21.2) |
| 2 points down | 12 | (23.1) |
| 3 points down | 5 | (9.6) |
| 4 points down | 3 | (5.8) |
| Total | 52 | (100.0) |

The majority (59.7 per cent) of those interviewed for the second time felt worse about their appearance than before surgery. Of these, by far the greatest number reported a score of one or two points lower than before.

The felt difference in appearance before and after surgery was compared between the two interviews, only for those 52 people interviewed for a second time. Table 9.51 compares the results for the two sets of interviews.

**Table 9.51**

**Felt Difference Between Before Surgery and Time of Interview - Comparison of First and Second Interviews     N = 52**

| At first interview | At second interview | | | | | | |
|---|---|---|---|---|---|---|---|
| | 1 pt. up | no diff. | 1 pt. down | 2 pt. down | 3 pt. down | 4pt. down | Total |
| No different | | 10 | 6 | 1 | | | 17 |
| 1 point down | 1 | 8 | | 4 | 2 | | 15 |
| 2 points down | | 1 | 3 | 5 | 1 | 1 | 11 |
| 3 points down | | 1 | 1 | 2 | 2 | 2 | 8 |
| 4 points down | | | 1 | | | | 1 |
| Total | 1 | 20 | 11 | 12 | 5 | 3 | 52 |

The significant differences shown are:

- Seven of those who had felt no different at first interview felt less positively about their appearance at second interview;

- Of the fifteen who had reported a one point deterioration at first interview, eight now rated their appearance one point higher, and six were less positive than before;

- Many of those who had scored two, three or four points lower at first interview had now improved their difference. The most marked was the person who had noted a four point difference between before illness and first interview; this person now only noted a one point difference.

A number of variables were then considered in relation to appearance, in order to see what influenced patients to reduce their rating of their appearance. In the next series of analyses, two aspects of appearance were examined. First, the variables were analysed in relation to felt difference at time of second interview, compared to how the person had felt about their appearance prior to surgery. Second, when these cross-tabulations had been completed, a further

266

analysis was carried out, relating the same variables to a further appearance variable, namely the difference between the changed view at first interview and the changed view of self at second interview. In this way, it was possible to see what contributed to patients' changed view of themselves between the two interviews.    Throughout this analysis, it must not be forgotten that the principal reason for changed feeling about the face could well be the changed face itself. In many instances, the contour was in fact altered, and residual scarring was frequent.    However, it is clear both from the literature and from observations in this study that the extent of acceptance of residual disfigurement is not necessarily related to the amount of the disfigurement itself. Hence it is important to see what other influences there are on acceptance in addition to the mutilation itself.

First, age was considered as an influence on changed view of appearance at second interview.    The results, which were not significant, did not present a clear pattern. What can be seen is that the three people whose view of their appearance had deteriorated most were those in the younger age bands, up to sixty. The one person who felt that things had improved was in his forties.

Gender was next considered as a possible factor influencing the acceptance of appearance. Table 9.52 describes the results of the analysis.

**Table 9.52**

**Gender and Felt Appearance (Second Interview)    N = 52**

(row percentages in brackets)

View of Own Appearance

|  | Down 4 pts. | Down 3 pts. | Down 2 pts | Down 1 pt. | Same | Up 1 pt. |
|---|---|---|---|---|---|---|
| Male | 2 | 4 | 5 | 6 | 14 | 1 |
|  | (6.2) | (12.5) | (15.6) | (18.8) | (43.8) | (3.1) |
| Female | 1 | 1 | 7 | 5 | 6 |  |
|  | (5.0) | (5.0) | (35.0) | (25.0) | (30.0) |  |
| Total | 3 | 5 | 12 | 11 | 20 | 1 |
|  | (5.8) | (9.6) | (23.1) | (21.2) | (38.5) | (1.9) |

More women than men had experienced reduced satisfaction with their appearance - 70 per cent compared to 53.1 per cent of men. Having said that, their dissatisfaction was at a moderate level, and more men appear at the extremes of three or four points reduced - 18.7 per cent compared to 10 per cent of women. The results were not significant.

The living situation of those interviewed for the second time was cross-tabulated to see what association it contained with variation in satisfaction with appearance. Table 9.53. describes this analysis.

**Table 9.53**
**Household Composition and Felt Appearance (Second Interview)**
**N = 52**
(row percentages in brackets)

View of Own Appearance

| | Down 4 pts. | Down 3 pts. | Down 2 pts | Down 1 pt. | Same | Up 1 pt. |
|---|---|---|---|---|---|---|
| Lives Alone | 1 (5.9) | 1 (5.9) | 5 (29.4) | 2 (11.8) | 8 (47.0) | nil |
| With Others | 2 (5.7) | 4 (11.4) | 7 (20.0) | 9 (25.7) | 12 (34.3) | 1 (2.8) |
| Total | 3 (5.8) | 5 (9.6) | 12 (23.1) | 11 (21.2) | 20 (38.5) | 1 (1.9) |

The results of this analysis, although not significant, suggest that those who live alone were less likely to have reduced their satisfaction with their own appearance than those who lived with a spouse or any another person. The difference is not overwhelming - 47 per cent of those who lived alone compared to 37.1 per cent of those who lived with others. For those whose satisfaction had reduced, little further clear pattern distinguished those who lived alone and those who lived with others.

The issue of social class and its association with changed view of appearance was then considered. Table 9.54 describes the results.

Table 9.54

**Social Class and Felt Appearance (Second Interview)**     **N = 52**
(row percentages in brackets)

View of Own Appearance

|  | Down 4 pts. | Down 3 pts. | Down 2 pts | Down 1 pt. | Same | Up 1 pt. |
|---|---|---|---|---|---|---|
| White Collar | 1 | 3 | 4 | 3 | 4 | nil |
|  | (6.7) | (20.0) | (26.7) | (20.0) | (26.7) |  |
| Manual | 2 | 2 | 8 | 8 | 16 | 1 |
|  | (5.4) | (5.4) | (21.6) | (21.6) | (43.2) | (2.7) |
| Total | 3 | 5 | 12 | 11 | 20 | 1 |
|  | (5.8) | (9.6) | (23.1) | (21.2) | (38.5) | (1.9) |

Although the results of this analysis were not significant, it can be seen that white collar patients were substantially more likely to have a reduced satisfaction with their own appearance by the time of the second interview - only 26.7 per cent of them stayed the same, contrasted with 45.9 per cent of manual patients who had either stayed the same or had improved their rating. Furthermore, the deterioration experienced by white collar patients was more likely to be a substantial one.

Patients had been asked whether in general terms they felt better at the time of interview than before surgery. The relationship between their responses and their changed feelings about their appearance was examined, and described in Table 9.55.

**Table 9.55**
**General Well-being and Felt Appearance (Second Interview)**
**N = 52**
(row percentages in brackets)

View of Own Appearance

|        | Down 4 pts. | Down 3 pts. | Down 2 pts | Down 1 pt. | Same | Up 1 pt. |
|--------|-------------|-------------|------------|------------|--------|----------|
| Better | nil | 1 | 8 | 5 | 8 | 1 |
|        |     | (4.3) | (34.8) | (21.7) | (34.8) | (4.3) |
| Same   | nil | 1 | 2 | 3 | 8 | nil |
|        |     | (7.1) | (14.3) | (21.4) | (57.1) | |
| Worse  | 3 | 3 | 2 | 3 | 4 | nil |
|        | (20.0) | (20.0) | (13.3) | (20.0) | (26.7) | |
| Total  | 3 | 5 | 12 | 11 | 20 | 1 |
|        | (5.8) | (9.6) | (23.1) | (21.2) | (38.5) | (1.9) |

The results did not quite reach significance (chi squared = 15.4 at a probability level of .11633), and the small numbers in most cells make interpretation difficult. However, there appeared to be a positive association between the two variables. In particular, those who felt generally the same as before surgery also tended to feel the same about their appearance. Those who felt worse generally tended to feel worse about their appearance than those who had a lower well- being score - 39.1 per cent felt the same or better, compared to 26.7 per cent of those who felt worse generally.

The composite "outlook" variable was next considered. Although it is essentially an outcome variable, a dependent variable, and has been used in this manner during the analysis, it was thought useful to see whether positive outlook was associated with a positive view of appearance. Outlook was considered in three ways. First, outlook at first interview was examined. The results of this cross- tabulation were not significant: those whose outlook had been moderate at first interview showed the least tendency to have reduced their satisfaction with their appearance, and those whose outlook had been low showed the greatest tendency. However, no clear trend is evident.

The previous analysis was concerned with outlook at first interview. Next, the association between outlook at second interview and felt difference about appearance was examined. The results, which were not significant, are reported in Table 9.56.

## Table 9.56
### Outlook (Second Interview) and Felt Appearance (Second Interview)    N = 52
(row percentages in brackets)

View of Own Appearance

|         | Worse      | Same       | Better    |
|---------|------------|------------|-----------|
| Low     | 2 (66.7)   | 1 (33.3)   | nil       |
| Medium  | 10 (71.4)  | 4 (28.6)   | nil       |
| High    | 19 (54.3)  | 15 (42.9)  | 1 (2.9)   |
|         |            |            |           |
| Total   | 31 (59.6)  | 20 (38.5)  | 1 (1.9)   |

Although the trend is not very clear, the figures suggest that improved outlook is associated with improved satisfaction with appearance.

The final stage in the process of relating outlook to appearance was to examine the difference between outlook at first interview and outlook at second, and to cross-tabulate the difference score with appearance. First, the association between change in outlook and changed view of appearance was considered. The results were not significant, and they were rather inconclusive. However, they suggested that those whose outlook had deteriorated had sustained a deterioration in their view of themselves; there was some slight suggestion that worsening of view of appearance was not as substantial for those whose outlook had stayed the same or had improved.

Moving to the next and final stage of consideration of changed appearance, the same series of variables were analysed to investigate their relationship with another aspect of changed view of appearance, namely the difference between the felt change at first interview and the felt change at second interview. Hence it was possible to see whether anything over and above the appearance itself affected individuals' adjustment to their changed appearance over a more substantial time after surgery. It must be remembered that during that time, facial appearance was likely to have improved objectively, because of the

271

healing of incisions and excisions, and the reduction of swelling caused by surgery. The appearance of the individual at second interview was nearer to what their longer term appearance was going to be.

In the first of these analyses, the age of the patient was related to difference in view of appearance between first and second interviews. Significance was not reached (chi squared $= 31.7$ at a probability level of .16763). Numbers are small, and so it is difficult to discern clear trends. Two points are worth noting: first, there is a large proportion of those in their fifties whose view of their appearance deteriorated - 77.8 per cent. Second, most of those in their sixties and seventies (82.8 per cent) had either the same view of their appearance or an improved view. All this must be set in the context that similar numbers overall were in each of the three categories of worse, the same or improved. The influence of gender on changed acceptance was considered next. Table 9.57 gives the results.

**Table 9.57**
**Gender and Changed Acceptance of Appearance  N = 52**

Changed Acceptance of Appearance

|  | Worse | Same | Better |
|---|---|---|---|
| Male | 2 (31.2) | 12 (37.5) | 10 (31.2) |
| Female | 7 (35.0) | 5 (25.0) | 4 (40.0) |
| Total | 17 (32.7) | 17 (32.7) | 18 (34.6) |

The distribution of scores for men was more even than that of women, most of whose scores had either deteriorated or improved, rather than remained the same. Forty per cent of women had improved their rating of their appearance. Having said that, the trends were not remarkable, and the results were not significant.

Next, living situation was examined for its relationship to changed view of appearance. The results are given in Table 9.58.

## Table 9.58
### Living Situation and Changed Acceptance of Appearance
### N = 52

Changed Acceptance of Appearance

|             | Worse       | Same        | Better      |
|-------------|-------------|-------------|-------------|
| Lives Alone | 5 (29.4)    | 4 (23.5)    | 8 (47.1)    |
| With Others | 12 (34.3)   | 13 (37.1)   | 10 (28.6)   |
| Total       | 17 (32.7)   | 17 (32.7)   | 18 (34.6)   |

The results were highly significant (chi squared = 36.4 at a probability level of .00007), and there was a strong suggestion that those who lived alone had improved their acceptance of their appearance since first interview.

The impact of social class was considered. The analysis is reported in Table 9.59.

## Table 9.59
### Social Class and Changed Acceptance of Appearance     N = 52

Changed Acceptance of Appearance

|              | Worse      | Same       | Better     |
|--------------|------------|------------|------------|
| White Collar | 7 (46.7)   | 5 (33.3)   | 3 (20.0)   |
| Manual       | 10 (27.0)  | 12 (32.4)  | 15 (40.5)  |
| Total        | 17 (32.7)  | 17 (32.7)  | 18 (34.6)  |

This analysis suggests (although the results were not significant) that white collar interviewees were less accepting of their revised appearance after the one year interval. Table 9.54 has already shown in its direct comparison between the point before surgery and the time of the second interview that white collar workers had a poorer view of their appearance than manual workers. The present table also shows that they had a poorer view than their view at first interview.

The general feeling of well-being of patients at second interview was next examined, and cross-tabulated with felt difference in acceptance of appearance. Table 9.60 gives the results.

**Table 9.60**
**General Well-being and Changed Acceptance of Appearance**
**N = 52**

Changed Acceptance of Appearance

|        | Worse      | Same       | Better      |
|--------|------------|------------|-------------|
| Better | 7 (30.4)   | 6 (26.1)   | 10 (43.5)   |
| Same   | 2 (14.3)   | 8 (57.1)   | 4 (28.6)    |
| Worse  | 8 (53 3)   | 3 (20.0)   | 4 (26.7)    |
| Total  | 17 (32.7)  | 17 (32.7)  | 18 (34.6)   |

The results were approaching significance (chi squared = 15.7 at a probability level of .10866), and a trend emerged whereby those who felt generally better now than before illness and surgery tended to have improved acceptance of their appearance.

The three measures of outlook were next considered for their relationship to changed acceptance of appearance; these were outlook at first interview, outlook at second interview, and the difference between the two. First, the association between outlook at first interview and change in acceptance of appearance was considered: although the pattern of results was uneven, generally it was towards the view that those whose outlook was low at first interview tended to have changed their view of their appearance for the worse between first and second interview.

The second outlook score, outlook at time of second interview, was cross-tabulated with change in acceptance of appearance. There was no clear pattern in the results, and they did not achieve significance.

Third, the difference between the two outlook scores was considered in relation to change in acceptance of appearance. This is reported in Table 9.61.

**Table 9.61**

**Change in Outlook (Between First and Second Interview) and
Changed Acceptance of Appearance     N = 52**

Changed Acceptance of Appearance

|          | Worse     | Same      | Better     |
|----------|-----------|-----------|------------|
| Outlook  |           |           |            |
| Lower    | 4 (57.1)  | 1 (14.3)  | 2 (28.6)   |
| Same     | 5 (62.5)  | 1 (12.5)  | 2 (25.0)   |
| Higher   | 8 (21.6)  | 15 (40.5) | 14 (37.8)  |
| Total    | 17 (32.7) | 17 (32.7) | 18 (34.6)  |

The results were approaching significance - chi squared = 7.6 at a probability level of .10485. They suggested that there was positive relationship between improved outlook score and improved acceptance of appearance.

**Appearance - a Summary**

By the time of the second interview, many people had changed their view of their appearance, for the better or the worse. The influence of a range of variables was considered in relation to the position at second interview. What is being described here is the change in the person's view of their appearance since before surgery began:

- There was little association between age and view of appearance at the time of second interview;

- More women than men had reduced their satisfaction with their appearance;

- Those who lived alone were less likely to have reduced satisfaction with appearance than those who lived with someone else;

- White collar workers tended to have reduced their satisfaction with their appearance more than manual workers;

- Those who felt better generally than before surgery also had a better view of their appearance;

- Improved outlook at second interview was associated with an improved view of appearance.

A further analysis was carried out, using the same variables, and relating them to the change in view of appearance between the first and second interviews:

- Several people in their fifties had poorer views of their appearance than at first interview, while most in their sixties and seventies tended towards an improved view of themselves;

- In the changed view of appearance between the two interviews, there was little difference between men and women;

- There was a highly significant suggestion that those who lived alone had improved their view of their own appearance more than those who lived with others;

- Manual workers were more accepting of their appearance after the year's interval;

- Those who felt better generally at second interview tended also to have changed their view of their appearance for the better;

- Outlook at first interview, and change in outlook between the interviews, had a positive association with changed view of appearance.

# 10 Testing the hypotheses

At the beginning of Part III, sixteen hypotheses were put forward. These hypotheses are now reviewed in the light of the empirical evidence.

1.  Patients with facial cancer will tend to be from the lower socio-economic groups, more male than female, in late middle age, and to be heavy smokers and drinkers. **Hypothesis supported**. The social characteristics of the sample were similar to those described in previous studies.

2.  Facially disfigured people will be stigmatised, and people will deal differently with those who have undergone facial surgery. **Hypothesis supported**. More than half the group felt that others' attitudes to them had changed for the worse. However, social contact and functioning were impaired more by the physical condition than by the attitudes of others.

3.  Patients will manage their differentness by 'covering', 'withdrawing' or 'fighting', to use Goffman's categories. **Hypothesis partially supported**. Withdrawal was observed to be the most common response.

4.  Patients will retain acceptance by those close to them, and will feel the greatest tension when meeting strangers. **Hypothesis partially supported**. Because of the tendency to withdraw, little contact with strangers took place. The little that did produce discomfort, particularly when children were encountered.

5.  Early detection of head and neck cancer will increase the

chances of survival. **Not capable of being tested without a longitudinal study.** Some social features associated with survival were beginning to emerge.

6.      Patients who are accepting of surgery and changed appearance will have a distinctive social profile. **Hypothesis supported.** Those who found it easier to accept the changes to themselves tended to be male, living alone, of manual occupation, and with strong egos.

7.      Patients will be assisted in their recovery by keeping control of their treatment and management. **Hypothesis untested.** Patients were largely passive recipients of treatment. This may have been due to the characteristics of the sample, or to the expectations of NHS patients in general.

8.      Patients will vary in the amount of reconstructive work which they feel they need, in order to satisfy their own self-respect, and to make them presentable to others. **Hypothesis supported.** Sometimes there was a strong motivation to improve appearance, and on other occasions patients were content that functional performance was restored.

9.      Patients who have had facial surgery are likely to experience feelings characteristic of bereavement, since changed facial appearance is a form of loss. **Hypothesis supported for a small number of patients.** The majority had been well prepared by the surgeons. On the other hand, most of the patients sustained a great loss because of reduced expectation of survival, and because of their reduced social functioning.

10.     Patients will feel separated from others because of difficulties with speech and eating, and because of their appearance. **Hypothesis supported.** Functional difficulties caused the greatest feelings of detachment, but fear of meeting people, particularly children, was noted.

11.     Surgery for head and neck cancer will be accompanied by signs of depression, dissatisfaction with the body, reduction in quality of life, and family tensions. **Hypothesis unproven.** Those whose outlook scores improved between the first and second interview tended to be living with others, of manual

occupations, and who felt that their appearance had not changed.

12. Patients who function better after illness and treatment will be those with strong and intact egos, older people with a settled way of life, and those with a good family support network. **Not supported**. Those who functioned best after surgery were female patients, living alone, and of white collar occupation. There was no association between feeling positive and functioning well.

13. Facial disfigurement through surgery will cause a major upheaval in people's lives. **Hypothesis supported**. The combined effect of the life- threatening condition, the painful and lengthy treatment, the residual scarring and functional deficit resulted in a substantial reduction in quality of life.

14. Good communication between surgeon and patient will enable trust to develop, which in turn will affect the patient's acceptance of surgery. **Hypothesis supported**. Where the surgeon was open with the patient, this was much appreciated.

15. Social workers will play a major part in the rehabilitation process. **Not supported**. Only a few patients had had any contact with a social worker, and this was for practical matters.

16. Patients will benefit from professional teamwork more than they would from professionals operating independently from each other. **Not proven**. Surgeons communicated well with each other, and surgeons and nurses worked in close co-operation, but there was little other sense of teamwork, and relatively little contact between hospital and community services.

# Conclusion

Facial disfigurement is associated with a distinctive set of difficulties, for the disfigured person, for the relatives and close associates of the disfigured person, and for professionals working in this field. In much of this study the emphasis has been on the needs and difficulties encountered by the disfigured person and his or her family; only to a limited extent have professional responses to these difficulties been considered so far. It was felt at the outset that social work in particular should have a part to play in responding to the social needs of those with a facial disfigurement, and in this concluding chapter the contribution of social work practice is examined.

In order to set this in context, brief reference is first made to the main point or lesson derived from each chapter in the study. Next, the social needs of those who undergo facial surgery are summarised. Then, ways in which social work can meet those needs are described, and this is followed by a discussion of the reasons why social workers have not assisted as much as their skills would suggest that they should. Finally, suggestions are made for improvements to services provided for disfigured people by social workers and others.

## Summary of the study

In the first four chapters, theoretical perspectives were presented. In Chapter One, through a sociological study of stigma it was shown that facially disfigured people have difficulty in managing their differentness, and that they need to adopt strategies to enable them to do so. In Chapter Two, a perspective was adopted which drew much from anthropology; from this it was evident that those with facial disfigurements encounter problems in their social relationships, and in establishing a stable social pattern of living for themselves. Chapter

Three, an analysis of the literary contributions of professionals in the field, contains a number of messages: the need for professionals to be sensitive to the vulnerabilities of the person who presents for treatment was emphasised, and so was the need for open communication between professionals. The social characteristics of disfigured people were described, and the impact of surgery and of disfigurement on their lives evaluated. The final chapter in the literature review, Chapter Four, contains lessons learned directly from people who have been disfigured. Points of particular stress are noted, together with ways in which those individuals have managed them.

The practice of a well-known plastic surgeon forms the basis for Chapter Five. Here too the value of openness and straightforwardness with patients is demonstrated. Next, it is shown in Chapter Six that groups of facially disfigured people can be of value to each other; they recognise the worth of each other, and together develop strategies for handling their differentness.

In Part III, Chapters Seven to Eleven, an empirical study is described. The results were strongly influenced by the nature of the available sample of patients who were treated for head and neck cancer: a clear profile emerged of ageing, working class men, whose expectations from life were modest; consequently, the impact of life-threatening illness and facial disfigurement was not as extreme as some of the literature would suggest it would have been. The most extreme impacts were experienced by those who diverged from this profile.

These are the principal lessons of the study. In the next section, some of these are considered in more detail, with special emphasis on those areas of need where social workers may be of help.


## Stresses encountered by facially disfigured people

*Facing the diagnosis*

An oral tumour is a very evident tumour, but it is frequently mistaken at its early stages for something less harmful. A lot of people did not pick it up for themselves. For these, a spouse, the dentist or G.P. first drew attention to it. Some patients, particularly men, were not very worried, or did not admit to being worried. This fits quite well with the cultural stereotype of the working-class male in northern industrial areas, where men have appeared stoical or indifferent about their health. (The Northern Health Region has a higher prevalence of head and neck cancer than the United Kingdom as a whole.) Is it hard to believe that one has such a tumour? One consultant described to the research staff a past patient with a tumour on the outside of her neck as big as an orange, which she said she had not noticed. Could it be a regionally differentiated phenomenon that people in the north-east, for example, report at a later stage than elsewhere? This requires further investigation; if strong denial is taking place, for cultural or any other reasons, this must be borne in mind by primary practitioners; dentists cannot, for example, rely on their patients to tell them that they are worried about a possible tumour, since the consequences of admission are too severe for the patients to tolerate.

*Time*

Waiting for treatment is a strain in itself, said by many to be the hardest thing to tolerate. Recovery from surgery is a slow process; reduction of swelling and healing of scars takes months, during which time great uncertainty exists for the patient and his or her family.

*Fear of recurrence*

This is a perfectly realistic fear, since the survival rate from head and neck cancer is poor. The chances of survival get better with every successive year, but the waiting is painful. If a person survives for one year, their chances of surviving long-term are 75 per cent, and if they survive for two years, the rate rises to 90 per cent.

The profile of those patients in the field study who survived up to the time of second interview is curious. If the profile is accurate or near to accurate, what does it mean, and can it be acted upon to any degree, and in any way? Are there social danger signals to which patients can respond by a variation in life style? It must be remembered that the relationship between social factors and survival is not causative, but associative, and it may be that a variation in life style is too late to avoid morbidity, once it has been established that a malignancy is present.

It is also unrealistic to assume that the factors which appear to be associated with survival are necessarily syndromic; possession of a cluster of them does not mean that the remainder will be present, or that survival is assured; however, it is interesting to summarise them: those who survive tend to be living alone, in the country, and smokers (the feature which runs counter to the epidemiological studies). They will be older women, in all likelihood middle class, who have had a good experience of treatment. Following treatment they will not have been over-exuberant, expressing neither extremes nor indifference to their appearance. Clearly this compilation of factors of which some are antecedent and others subsequent is not a reliable approach, and what is called for is a collaborative study between social scientist and clinician, which might produce useful and reliable social indicators of clinical risk.

## Appearance

In addition to actual survival, for many there is fear about long-term appearance. It will be difficult to determine initially how much scarring will be permanent. The study also showed that the actual extent of disfigurement does not determine the extent of psychological discomfort. So the fear of long-term disfigurement is a realistic feature for all who undergo facial surgery.

Fear of disfigurement and dislike of one's new appearance is one consequence of changed appearance. The other is discomfort and difficulty in relating to others. Where those others are close relatives and friends, to whom one's appearance is only one aspect of knowing the individual, changed appearance may be of lesser consequence. Many of the people in the empirical study were restricted in their opportunities for new encounters, which minimised any attendant discomfort. Those who did have significant encounters with relative strangers described awkwardness and distress.

## Which treatment?

There is on occasions a social component in deciding a preferred course of treatment. In most instances, clinical factors will determine whether radiotherapy or surgery (or both) should be pursued. However, clinicians sometimes need to consider the tolerance and resilience of the individual to the stresses engendered by each form of treatment. Social or psychological aspects may influence a decision on the type or extent of treatment, and in this social workers should see two tasks for them - to assist in the assessment of the strengths and qualities of the individual, and to help that person to express a preference when it is realistic that they should do so.

## Family disruption

The extent of family disruption occasioned by surgery is hard to anticipate. However, all patients and their families may certainly expect a minimum of disturbance, which will affect the individuals and their collective functioning: at very least there will be separation, fear for the family member who is the patient, the physical wear and tear on the patient, and the fatigue of visiting him or her while keeping the remainder of the household functioning, uncertainty about the extent of recovery, and adjustment of role because of the increased dependency of the ill person.

Whether more serious damage is caused to relationships and family functioning is likely to depend on the existing strengths within the family. Many patients reported that their relationship with their spouse had improved since surgery. The literature tells us that such people are likely to have had sound relationships in the first place. Those most at risk are those whose foundations were not so solid. There is a danger in any loss sustained by a family of that family moving apart. Consequently, professionals must be alert to those vulnerable people who are most likely to be affected by the impact of changed appearance and reduced functioning.

*Functional impairment*

Patients and their families must be warned about difficulties with speaking and eating which they are likely to encounter. Such difficulties are painful, distressing, problematic in a practical way, and most isolating. They need to be aware that some of the problems will go away over time, but residual speech difficulties require and can be helped by speech therapy. The more immediate eating difficulties may be assisted by the advice of a dietician. Patients need to know that such help will be available.

Head and neck surgery also results in functional impairment of other parts of the body; when a graft is used in order to reconstruct the face, the site from which it is taken often suffers. If a piece of bone from the hip is used, walking is made more difficult, at least temporarily. If skin and tissue are taken from the chest, the tissue that remains is stretched to make good the gap. This means that full flexion of the arm is made difficult, sometimes permanently. Thus the difficulties which result from facial surgery can reach far beyond the face to include general mobility and self-care problems.

*Isolation*

The isolation occasioned by difficulties with eating and speaking has already been described. Fear for the future and discomfort over changed appearance make going home from hospital a worrying time, and patients need to be reassured that they are not going to be abandoned by the caring establishment in which so much has happened to them: their appearance has been changed, their life-threatening illness has been treated, they may have acquired a new disfigurement through the surgical process. The hospital is a safe place, containing caring people who have been of value to patients. The links must in some way be maintained after discharge. Otherwise, as was found in the empirical study, strong feelings of isolation are experienced.

*Finance*

Finance is likely to produce difficulties for those who undergo such a process of treatment, although it may not be any more acute an issue for the group being considered than for any other patient group. Nonetheless it may be helpful if patients are reminded of the financial stress which they might incur, and if they are given help to reduce its impact - advice on welfare benefits, grants from voluntary agencies, and general financial management advice.

*Power and powerlessness*

Most of those who featured in the field study were poor and relatively inarticulate people; the impression was formed that they had a passive attitude to illness, and to their power over how it was treated. The surgeon is a very powerful person, and the patient and family may need help in expressing their views and opinions about the treatment process. They may feel diffident about enquiring about the process of treatment and its pacing, and questions about future treatment - choice of treatment, and whether to undergo further reconstructive work. Most of the surgeons whom I met were, from my perspective, compassionate, approachable people, but it may still be the case that the individual patient needs someone else who can act as their advocate, however benign and non-adversarial the circumstances. The most able and strong person can feel vulnerable when undergoing medical treatment. Such vulnerability will be heightened if the face is affected, since this may alter the composure needed to meet new and difficult situations.

*Emotional and functional well-being*

The empirical study suggested that a positive emotional state did not automatically result in enhanced functioning. It would be fruitless to argue for one or the other being more important: this will differ from person to person. In any case, there is no suggestion that the individual or the therapist has any influence on which aspect to emphasise for any individual. Rather, they are being highlighted as two distinct areas, which need to be appraised separately, and worked on separately. Each individual will know which is more important to them: to feel good, or to function well. It is not possible to prepare people completely for such an upheaval in their lives, since the extent of upheaval is not known until after the event, and will depend on the strengths and supports of the individual, but awareness of the issues described above may help to offset the shock which they experience. It was with this end in view that the staff of Sunderland Oral and Maxillo-Facial Surgery Department and I compiled the video already referred to, which is included as Appendix II. However, this is only a small component of what is needed. What will be suggested in the next section is that social work has a particularly significant part to play in assisting individuals and their families in tolerating the stresses likely to be engendered by facial disfigurement and surgery, and in adjusting to changed appearance, role and functioning.

## The contribution of social work

When patients were asked in the field study when help and support were most needed, they gave clear indicators that they welcomed close contact with the treatment centre, particularly after the acute phase was over. The interviewers frequently found that the research interviewer was seized on as providing the first opportunity which the patients and their carers had to speak about how stressful the experience had been. When the writer rang one family to obtain permission for the interviewer to visit, the patient's wife said "Thank God you've called. There's been no one to talk to about how dreadful it's been." The interviewers found that they had to absorb some of the feelings resulting from the illness and treatment, for the patients themselves, and for their families, particularly for their spouses. The interviewers were all trained social workers, and were able to do so appropriately without deflecting their efforts too far from the research task. The point is that they kept receiving messages about the needs of the families - requests to call again when passing, and certainly not to wait a year before visiting again (for the second interview). A few families were referred to social work agencies for help, where the focus for intervention was sufficiently precise. Of the remainder a few were mentioned to the surgeon, if the patient had consented to this.

The consultant surgeon most actively involved in the study agreed to participate because he wanted to learn how better to provide social support for his patients. He was on the point of recruiting a nurse counsellor when the study began, but decided to hold back until at least some of the results of the study were available to him. The results show that few people other than clinical and nursing staff provide help around the time of treatment, in addition to the actual treatment. Surgeons were the most helpful, providing information or advice in many cases. They also provided a "listening" service for 13 people. Few people saw any professional as providing a counselling service. This may be because no one did, or because what was provided was not recognised as counselling.

Whereas surgeons and nurses (and to a smaller degree general practitioners) provided the professional help, be it information or advice or listening, social workers and ministers, the traditional sympathetic advisers and listeners, featured scarcely at all.

It may be that surgeons find personal counselling a fulfilling and important task. Indeed they were identified within the study as the professionals most involved with counselling and support. Yet there are three strong reasons why such a task should not be left to them. First, their job is to practise surgery; they are a scarce and expensive resource, and rightly spend a large proportion of their time in the operating theatre. Second, they are not trained in counselling techniques: this is not where their skills lie. Finally, patients in the study made it clear that they needed professional support and counselling long after the acute stage of illness was over. Surgeons are unlikely to be available for this, since their priority must be those in acute need of surgery.

In the remainder of this chapter, the role of social workers in helping disfigured persons is considered; first, ways in which social workers can be of value are summarised; the counselling role is described in slightly more detail. Second, reasons for the failure of social work to respond to the challenge of facial disfigurement are suggested. Finally, ways of enhancing services for disfigured people are proposed.

*Social work and facial disfigurement*

There are indeed six possible roles for the social worker in the context of facial disfigurement; these roles are general social work roles, but all appropriate to this particular area of need:

1.    Assessment

Two forms of assessment have relevance here:   first, the social worker may carry out an assessment as a contribution to a decision-making process - in this context the decision-making process might be whether and how to proceed with treatment. There are parallels with the compilation of social reports for a range of purposes, such as court hearings or school allocation panels, at the request, for example, of a parent, a court, or an adoption panel. The social worker may participate in the screening process, to decide whether surgery should be undertaken. Where possible, this should be a participative process, rather than an excluding, esoteric judgement on the patient's capacity. In this way the patient may be helped towards an understanding of what is possible and what is not possible in the context. This role will apply both to surgery for congenital deformity and to operations for the excision of malignancy. In the latter case, screening may contribute to choices of treatment, and to decisions on whether to proceed with further reconstructive work. Whoever conducts the screening process (and ideally it should be a team approach), the literature makes it clear that openness will produce the best results and the least dissatisfaction.

The second sense in which assessment could be valuable within the context of on-going social casework or counselling. In this sense assessment is not a discrete exercise, but an integral element of a special relationship: practitioner and helped come together to agree common grounds for working, a common objective, and an allocation of tasks. The earliest reference to the assessment process is in Mary Richmond's "Social Diagnosis,"[1] but as Perlman pointed out, it was unrealistic of Mary Richmond to have seen diagnosis as a separate preliminary task:

> One difficulty was that clients would not stand still while the study was being made; another was that they would not always see eye to eye with the caseworker in the treatment plan that careful diagnosis prescribed.[2]

Rather, it should be seen as an element in the process of engaging in a contract with each other:

> Problems perceived by the client are elicited, explored, and clarified by the caseworker in the initial interview. The problem which the client is most anxious to resolve is normally

seen as the primary target of intervention, if it meets the criteria of the model. If the client does not acknowledge a problem that would provide an acceptable target of intervention, the practitioner attempts to determine if one is present through a systematic review with the client of possible problem areas.[3]

It would be proper for the social worker to engage in a process of joint assessment with the facial surgery patient, in order to determine whether there was an agreed need for social work help, which would take any of the following five forms.

## 2.    Resource brokerage

The need was expressed several times during the empirical study for clear information about a range of resources - access to additional nursing, financial advice, membership of mutual help groups, addresses of support groups. This is a straightforward, simple task, which must not be overlooked. The social worker as broker should be well acquainted with local and national resources, and ensure that information about them is communicated to patients at as early a stage as possible.

## 3.    Advocacy

The social worker has a clear part to play in assisting the patient and family to speak out about their needs, preferences and choices. It has already been acknowledged that for a number of reasons people with a facial disfigurement may not be very powerful people. Without being strident, the social work member of the professional team has the ability to articulate the requirements and views of those who are inhibited from doing so by the power relationship implicit within clinical and social work practice.

## 4.    Linking with the hospital

The social worker can offer a range of constructive means to reduce the isolation felt by virtually all patients who undergo facial surgery. This is not necessarily isolation from the community in which they live, but rather a feeling of severance from the hospital, when acute treatment is over. The social worker attached to the clinical team may be the professional responsible for maintaining the link between patient and hospital, until reduction of clinical need and resumption of normal life make the need for such a link less urgent.

## 5.    Groupwork

A clear role has been established for professionals to assist in the establishment and running of mutual help groups. Some of these are facilitated by nurses, some by occupational therapists, and others by social workers. Group work of a variety of forms comes well within the competence of social workers, and they have a clear part to play. The profile of the social worker within the group will vary according to its aims and according to the skills and wishes of the other participants. The extent of the social worker's influence in the group would be negotiated with the group.

## 6.    Counselling

"Counselling" is a widely-used and often misused expression. It is frequently used by clinicians to mean the imparting of clinical information, which may then be used by the patient to inform their choice about future treatment. This is an extremely restricted use of the term, although the context in which the clinician imparts such information might well be one where counselling is indicated. In this section, a model is proposed for counselling people with a facial disfigurement, drawing on social work theory, deviance theory and psycho-dynamic theory. The framework is not described in all its detail, since all that is intended is to demonstrate that it is reasonable for social workers to contribute in this area, supported by a sound knowledge-base.

Properly applied, the term "counselling" will always be supported by a model of explanation of human behaviour, be it psycho-dynamic theory, systems theory, or a behavioural approach. Using psycho-dynamic theory as an illustration, it can be said that counselling is a progressive relationship which develops between the counsellor and individual. In this the counsellor draws upon acquired theoretical knowledge and personal awareness, in order to enhance the person's perception and understanding of his or her particular problems. Great emphasis is placed on the influence of early life experiences, especially those unresolved negative experiences which then affect the feelings and thoughts of the adult.

Although counselling need not necessarily be defined in these terms, such a definition offers a useful framework for practice: it is a person-centred, analytical approach that encourages self-awareness in the individual to a particular area of his or her life which is causing concern. Consequently, not only is the individual assisted with the immediate problem, but he or she can learn, as Sainsbury says, to expand

> ....his understanding of the personal and social resources available to him, and in strengthening his ability to use these resources to satisfy both his own needs and the expectations of others concerning his behaviour.[4]

The counsellor acts as a medium by which the person learns to moderate and regulate the conflicting demands of social relationships and personal tensions. The therapeutic relationship works towards the

> ....realistic goal of achieving some restored or new equilibrium.[5]

The relationship is not a normal social relationship, and it requires commitment on both sides to a process which can be taxing and distressing. If the person is going to feel able to reveal and unburden himself or herself of intimate, stressful feelings, the counsellor needs to be someone who can withstand the impact of the disclosures, and to be strong enough to endure the intensity of the emotions which are expressed. The counsellor must be both resilient and receptive.

In dealing with facial disfigurement, the counsellor must be aware of the possible impact on the individual of congenital or acquired disfigurement. There must also be an awareness of strategies for adjusting to disfigurement - by the disfigured person and by others. One such framework is offered by Davis, who describes the process of managing the discomfort generated by disfigurement, which he calls "deviance disavowal."[6]

Davis describes three stages through which the disfigured person may pass, before a comfortable relationship may be established with another person. He is referring to the middle range of social relationships - not the passing of the time of day, and not the closest relationships, but those where some significant engagement must occur. The first phase, known as "fictional acceptance," requires some denial of the issue which is occupying the minds of both parties in the encounter, namely the disfigurement. This is necessary to make progress with the relationship, but it is also hazardous, since the encounter may never proceed beyond this superficial level.

In the next phase, "breaking through," the disfigured person helps the other to become comfortable with him or her, raising the normal aspects of profile, and reducing the emphasis on abnormality, through a number of strategies.

> These range from relatively straightforward conversational offerings in which he alludes in passing to his involvement in a normal round of activities, to such forms of indirection as interjecting taboo or privatised references by way of letting the normal know that he does not take offence at the latter's uneasiness or regard it as a fixed obstacle to achieving rapport.[7]

When entry has been gained in this way, it is then necessary to sustain it; this (third) stage is known as "institutionalising the normalised relationship."

> Having disavowed deviance and induced the other to respond to him as he would to a normal, the problem then becomes one of sustaining the normalised definition in the face of the many small amendments and qualifications that must frequently be made to it.[8]

Within a general framework of counselling, the social worker may also offer this framework of "deviance disavowal" to the disfigured person (or to those who work or live with disfigured people) as a means of adjustment and growth. Counselling will involve reflection on the stages of adjustment, where necessary interpreting the behaviour of the individual or that of others, and relating it to Davis' model. Where learning through insightful reflection is not a practical option, role play between individual and counsellor may be a useful alternative.

Facial disfigurement is loss - loss of the face previously known and accepted, by the individual and by others. The social worker plays a part in helping the person adjust to this loss, which in some ways may take the individual through the same stages of adjustment as those experienced by the bereaved person. The process of healthy mourning has, as a general premise, the proposal that the bereaved individual aims to withdraw emotional investment in the deceased, and to reinvest it in other relationships, thereby filling the space created by that death. Within this there are infinite variations, since each bereavement, and each mourning, is unique. Bowlby defines mourning as:

A fairly wide array of psychological processes set in train by the loss of a loved person, irrespective of their outcome.[9]

and grieving as:

The condition of a person who is experiencing the distress at loss and experiencing it in a more or less overt way.[10]

Throughout his work in this area he emphasises the multiplicity of personal and environmental factors affecting bereavement reactions; consequently the possible grief patterns are virtually limitless. Parkes states:

No two griefs are the same and 'solutions' that work for one person may not work for another.[11]

He is working within a medical model, which views bereavement as a 'syndrome' or cluster of grief symptoms. These include somatic distress, pre-occupation and general physical dysfunction. Thus bereavement is defined in terms of a pathological disorder, which needs to be treated. This is not a positive view of human behaviour, and may not always be helpful. What is helpful, however, is Parkes' analysis of grief and mourning, which is based upon this model.

He proposes that there are four stages to grief, and that the bereaved person needs to pass through these before a healthy resolution can be achieved. This suggests a rather passive process, which will maintain its own momentum. Worden[12] proposes a much more active model of grief, a dynamic involvement of the bereaved person with the 'tasks' of grief, which he defines as:

Task 1:     To accept the reality of the loss;
Task 2:     To experience the pain of grief;
Task 3:     To adjust to an environment in which the deceased is missing;
Task 4:     To withdraw emotional energy and invest it in another relationship.

Only after completion of task one can the bereaved person move on to the other three tasks, not necessarily in linear order, but with frequent oscillations back and forth between them.

In order to achieve completion of the tasks of mourning, the individual must invest vast resources of physical, cognitive and emotional energy. Hence bereaved persons often complain of exhaustion while being unable to sleep.

The application of this process to the social work task with facially disfigured people is in a sense addressed by Parkes, who explains how

> ....some of the phenomena that have emerged in studies of the reaction to bereavement are found in similar form following other types of loss.[13]

Consequently, much of the counselling approach used in bereavement counselling is also applicable to counselling people who are facially disfigured. In addition, many who undergo facial disfigurement are aware in advance of its likelihood. An opportunity therefore exists for adequate preparation:

> Any plan for change should include an attempt to understand and provide for the psychosocial effects of the change. Thus the decision to remove a leg should be made in full awareness of the patient's prospects of making a successful adjustment to life as an amputee; plans for slum clearance should be made in full awareness of the probable effects of relocation upon the population to be resettled.[14]

The concept applies equally to those about to undergo facial surgery. Sufficient knowledge now exists of the likely consequences of the procedure, and of the best means of adjusting to it. It falls to the social worker to apply the knowledge in their practice.

The framework for practice is therefore three-fold: within general social work theory, two further strands are present. One helps understand how individuals overcome loss, and re-invest in a newly-shaped world, which in this case includes a newly-shaped face. The other helps explain how people learn to behave with others when they have acquired a revised facial appearance, and how others adapt to them. Both these resources, when used within the context of social work theory, will enrich it and make it more relevant to the specialist setting of facial surgery.

*The failure of social work*

The approach to counselling described in the previous section is by no means new - it is one of many widely-accepted ways of responding to need, disadvantage and loss. However, it has been shown in this study that social workers do not contribute substantially to the support of people who have undergone facial surgery. The need is clear, the skills exist which could meet the need; why do social workers do so little to help? In this section, a number of possible explanations are given. It is suggested that they have all contributed to the failure of social work to help in this context.

*Social work education*

With the development of generic social work came generic social work education. Medical social workers no longer underwent a separate, specialist process of education, and the proportion of general social work education allotted to hospital social work issues is not substantial. Working with ill people is not seen as a priority. Social work tutors might argue that they are simply reflecting the priorities and pressures of the profession.

*Statutory requirements*

Certain social work tasks, particularly those related to child protection and care, are circumscribed by elaborate legislation and regulations. For many local authority social services and social work departments, there is little scope for pursuing work other than that required by statute. The Children Act 1989, recognised as the most powerful instrument of child protection ever enacted, also places substantially increased demands on the resources of authorities.

*Inquiries*

The effect of successive inquiries into child death through abuse has been to construct elaborate procedures for the protection of children thought to be at risk of abuse. In both the Rochdale and the Orkney inquiries it has been clear that authorities were expected to learn lessons from previous investigations (in those instances the Cleveland experience was cited). Consequently, large proportions of local authority resources are dedicated to ensuring the protection of children and families, and also of communities and of professional staff. These resources might otherwise have been distributed more evenly within departments, and allocated to areas where questions of authority and statute are less of an issue.

*Successful intervention*

It is reasonable that professionals should devote the majority of their time to areas of work which are going to produce success, and minimise the time dedicated to work which has a high likelihood of failure. It could be argued that since the primary condition of facial disfigurement is not going to be ameliorated by social workers, they should not devote much time to helping those with such a condition. Instead, they are better employed in family preventive work, arranging alternative care for those who cannot be cared for within their own families, and sustaining it by careful supervision - a form of social triage. Such an analysis is questionable; social workers cannot eliminate the disfigurement, but they can do much to reduce its social and emotional impact.

*Stigma by association*

If facially disfigured people are stigmatised, so might be those who associate with them. To befriend someone who is stigmatised is to risk the same stigma adhering to one. This may be the view of some social workers.

*The hidden nature of the problem*

Most of the suggested reasons for the failure of social work to respond to this issue assume that a conscious choice has been made not to respond. However, it is likely that many social workers, and the managers of the resources of departments, are unaware either of the nature or of the extent of the problem. They have not helped because they have been unaware that there was an issue.

*The organisational context*

The most likely setting for the social worker who will provide a specialist service to facial surgery patients is within the hospital itself. Although community-based social workers may express an interest and on occasions respond to expressed need, they are unlikely to encounter the phenomena with sufficient frequency and in sufficient numbers to enable them to develop the skills needed to be of most help. At the time of writing this conclusion (Summer 1991), hospital social work in the United Kingdom is under considerable scrutiny, which at times threatens its professionalism, and its future existence as a separate specialism is in question. Five distinct influences can be identified: first, local authorities are, not for the first time, experiencing severe financial difficulties; a recent variation on this long- standing issue is the added burden imposed by community charge defaulting. Second, the fact that both health authorities and local authorities are engaging in more explicit contractual relationships with each other and with other agencies has thrown into question the previously less formal secondment of social workers from local authorities to health authorities. Social services and social work departments may start charging for the service, and health boards and authorities may decide that they cannot or will not afford it. Third, there is considerable public, political and professional pressure on social work agencies, already referred to, to enhance their child protection services, and this may be at some cost to other services. Fourth, legislation has been enacted, likely to be implemented in 1993, which places the locus of care firmly in the community. Finally, hospital social workers have not always promoted themselves and their models of practice with the vigour necessary to convince their colleagues, managers and the public of their unique contribution to professional practice.

## Services for disfigured people

Social workers and their managers may recognise that they can help disfigured people, but competition for scarce resources remains an issue. It may be that, because of the greater awareness of the problems faced by disfigured people brought about by individuals who have written about their experience, those in control of resources become more disposed to assist. It is also hoped that this study contributes to that process. However, it must be acknowledged that in a period of diminishing services, much re-allocation of social work time in this direction is unlikely. The best that may be obtained is for the issue to be tabled for consideration when the economic difficulties of local government are alleviated.

Meanwhile, further possibilities could be explored:

1.  In some areas of hospital social work, voluntary funding of social work posts has been obtained, which is allocated to a very specific area of specialism (children's cancer, cystic fibrosis, kidney patients, for example). This is normally achieved through close co-operation between local authority staff and voluntary organisations. If any such funding were to be obtained, it would also be heavily dependent for its

successful use on close collaboration with surgical staff;

2.  Teamwork between professionals was emphasised in the literature. It becomes even more important, if the social work role is to be enhanced, that trust should be established between the surgeon, nurse and social worker, so that each can be clear when they are the most appropriate professional to engage the patient in dialogue;

3.  Counselling courses for surgeons - if surgeons feel that they have a part to play in counselling disfigured people, should they be helped to do so by the provision of counselling courses? This would be a positive and pragmatic response - surgeons feel that they do and should counsel, so train them to do so. Such training would either enhance their skills or show them that they do not have the time to counsel effectively. At very least such an experience would enhance their communication skills, which were found in the literature to be related to acceptance of the results of surgery;

4.  At the Mayo Clinic, a staff-member known as the nurse educator offered advice to patients on how to manage their altered physical state - how to handle a prosthesis, what to expect the altered body to look like, and what to do as a consequence. In many respects, this role is fulfilled by the out patient sister in British hospitals. The further development of this role could be considered. Again, training in counselling could be offered on a broader basis (some out-patient sisters are already trained in counselling);

5.  Groupwork has been shown to be effective for many as a means of feeling accepted and cared for, of feeling understood and valued. While not providing the solution for everyone, groups could be made more widely available, with greater support from clinicians, nurses, social workers and health service managers. It has been suggested in this study that local groups are unlikely to flourish without professional backing. When they do receive such support, they become a strong component of the individual's response to their condition. If they were to become a major resource, they would require greater backing from health service managers, in order to enhance the contribution made by voluntary effort.

In this chapter emphasis has been placed on the role of the social worker and other professionals in working with people with a facial disfigurement. However, it must be emphasised that none of these processes should be seen in isolation. The literature suggests that only through efficient team work can a complete and satisfactory service be provided to the patient undergoing facial surgery. Team work is expensive, time-consuming and difficult; it is often the element which gets forgotten by busy people, but the communication which it implies is the single most important theme running throughout this study - communication between doctor and patient (Frances Macgregor), between professionals (Ian Munro), between groups of patients (Archibald McIndoe), and, most crucially, between patients and those close to them (Christine Piff). A crisis may bind people together, but at least as frequently it drives them apart, be they patients, professionals, or a combination of the two. A centripetal input is required to counteract such a centrifugal force, to which all those associated with the phenomenon of facial disfigurement are susceptible. In this study the impact of distortion of appearance has been examined, and ways of minimising it explored. This is a crucial task, since the association between face and human feelings and behaviour is fundamental, and distortion of the face is to put at risk the individual's full participation in life.

**Notes**

1.  Richmond, M., 1922, *What is Social Casework?*, Russell SageFoundation, New York
2.  Perlman, H.H., 1957, Social Casework, a Problem-solving Process University of Chicago Press, Chicago, p. viii.
3.  Reid, W.J. and Epstein, L., 1972, *Task-Centred Casework*, Columbia Press, New York, p. 21.
4.  Sainsbury, E., 1973, *Social Diagnosis in Casework*, Routledge and Kegan Paul, London, p. 74.
5.  Reid, W.J. and Shyne, A., 1970, *Brief and Extended Casework*, Columbia Press, New York, p. vi.
6.  Davis, F., 1961-2, 'Deviance Disavowal: the Management of Strained Interaction by the Visibly Handicapped,' *Social Problems*, 9, pp. 120-132.
7.  op. cit., p. 128.
8.  op. cit., p. 130.

9.  Bowlby, J., 1981, 'Attachment and Loss: Vol. III', *Loss: Sadness and Depression*, Penguin, Harmondsworth, p. 17.
10. op. cit., p. 18.
11. Worden, J.W., 1983, *Grief Counselling and Grief Therapy*, Tavistock, London and New York, p. ix.
12. op. cit.
13. Parkes, C.M., 1975, *Bereavement: Studies of Grief in Adult Life*, Penguin, Harmondsworth. p.223.
14. op. cit., p. 225.

# Appendix 1:
# Interview schedules

**Facial surgery study**

First interview

1.    Reference Number:

2.    Age:

3.    Sex:

4.    Occupation (or occupation before retirement):

5.    Area of Residence:    Urban        [  ]
                            Suburban     [  ]
                            Rural        [  ]

6.    Lives with:    Spouse/partner    [  ]
                     Parent(s)         [  ]
                     Child(ren)        [  ]
                     Other rel.        [  ]
                     Non-rel.          [  ]
                     Alone             [  ]

7.  Social Class:     Professional          [  ]
                      Intermediate          [  ]
                      Skilled non-m.        [  ]
                      Skilled man           [  ]
                      Part-skilled m.       [  ]
                      Unskilled man.        [  ]
                      Looking after home    [  ]

8.  Name or describe the six people whom the interviewee sees most often, and say how long ago they were last seen.

|   | Name/description | How long ago seen |
|---|------------------|-------------------|
| 1 |                  |                   |
| 2 |                  |                   |
| 3 |                  |                   |
| 4 |                  |                   |
| 5 |                  |                   |
| 6 |                  |                   |

9.  How long ago did interviewee last go out shopping?

10. How long ago did interviewee last work?

11. How long ago did interviewee go out to any outside entertainment (e.g. cinema)?

12. How long before surgery/treatment did condition exist?

13. How long before surgery/treatment was patient worried about it?

14. How long was it before patient communicated concern to someone else?

15. Comments:

16. Who identified the fact that the interviewee had a problem? (e.g. self, spouse, clinician)

17. What was wrong - full description of interviewee's understanding at the start:

18. What was the doctor's diagnosis?

19. What did the surgeons/physicians do? Describe the process - more than one treatment episode if relevant:

20. Is any further treatment anticipated?

21. Was treatment successful?

22. Although it is early to say, does interviewee feel better or worse than before treatment?

|               |     |
|---------------|-----|
| Better        | [ ] |
| About the same | [ ] |
| Worse         | [ ] |

23. Does interviewee see more or less people than before surgery?

|               |     |
|---------------|-----|
| Less          | [ ] |
| About the same | [ ] |
| More          | [ ] |

24. Is there any change in employment status?

| | | |
|---|---|---|
| Lost job | [ | ] |
| Gained job | [ | ] |
| Promotion | [ | ] |
| Demotion | [ | ] |
| Same job | [ | ] |
| Similar job | [ | ] |
| Unemp. thr'out | [ | ] |
| Not known | [ | ] |

25. Financial situation since illness:

a.
| | | |
|---|---|---|
| Income up | [ | ] |
| Income same | [ | ] |
| Income down | [ | ] |

b.
| | | |
|---|---|---|
| Expenditure up | [ | ] |
| Expend. same | [ | ] |
| Expend. down | [ | ] |

26. Estimate the cost of additional items of expenditure:

27. Are there any leisure activities which were enjoyed before treatment which interviewee is now unable to follow? Give details:

28. Comment on any major change in any of the following aspects of life:

a. house

b. friends

c. religious observances

29.    Estimate of interviewee's satisfaction with life:

    a.                Enthusiastic      [ ]

                                                [ ]

                                              [ ]

                                              [ ]

                Apathetic         [ ]

    b.                Fulfilled         [ ]

                                                [ ]

                                              [ ]

                                              [ ]

                Missed chances  [ ]

    c.                Optimistic      [ ]

                                              [ ]

                                              [ ]

                                              [ ]

                Pessimistic      [ ]

30.    Are these findings related to illness/surgery or to other factors?

31.    Estimate of level of functioning since onset of illness:

    a.    Relations with spouse/closest other:

                Better            [ ]

                About the same   [ ]

                Worse            [ ]

    b.    Relations with other household members (if any):

                Better            [ ]

                About the same   [ ]

                Worse            [ ]

c.      Carrying out home responsibilities:

            Better             [ ]
            About the same   [ ]
            Worse             [ ]

d.      Work performance (if employed):

             Better             [ ]
            About the same   [ ]
            Worse             [ ]

e.      Financial situation:

             Better             [ ]
            About the same   [ ]
            Worse             [ ]

f.      Satisfaction with living environment:

             Better             [ ]
            About the same   [ ]
            Worse             [ ]

g.      Making use of community resources (e.g. library, park, etc.)

             Better             [ ]
            About the same   [ ]
            Worse             [ ]

32.    General satisfaction with past appearance:

             Perf. content     [ ]
            Quite content    [ ]
            Indifferent      [ ]
            Dislike          [ ]
            Hate              [ ]

33. General satisfaction with present appearance:

| | |
|---|---|
| Perf. content | [  ] |
| Quite content | [  ] |
| Indifferent | [  ] |
| Dislike | [  ] |
| Hate | [  ] |

34. Because of changed appearance (if any), does interviewee think that people have changed in their attitude to him/her?

| | |
|---|---|
| Yes | [  ] |
| No | [  ] |

35. Describe who has changed, and in what way:

36. How long was interviewee's last stay in hospital?

37. Description of life in hospital, staff attitudes, own feelings, attitudes to therapy, etc.

38. Describe who was helpful during illness and treatment, and in what way?

39. Do you have any suggestions for improved services from these or any other people?

Surgeon
Other clinician
Psychiatrist
G.P.
Priest/minister
Max.fac. technician
Social worker
Psychologist
Union Rep.

Voluntary Group
Friends/Relatives

40a.   When is/was help needed? (more than one if relevant)

                        At diagnosis          [  ]
                        Pre-op.               [  ]
                        Post-op.              [  ]

40b.   Comments:

41.    Comments on smoking habits:

42.    Earlier episodes in hospital (for whatever the reason):

43.    Other family members' history of morbidity:

44.    What has been the worst thing of all?

45.    Would interviewee be happy to be interviewed again in twelve
       months?

46.    Additional comments:

47.    Interviewed alone or with other:

48.    If with another, with whom?

49.    Time spent on interview:

50.    Date of interview:

51.    Interviewer:

52.    Date report written:

# Bibliography

Addison, C., 1975, 'Social aspects of facial prosthetics,' *International Prosthetic Workshop, Part I,* Institute of Maxillo-facial Technology, pp. 146-152.

Arndt, E.M., Travis, F., Lefebvre, A., Nice, A. and Munro, I.R., 1986,'Beauty and the eye of the beholder: social consequences and personal adjustment of facial patients', *British Journal of Plastic Surgery,* 39, pp. 81-84,

Arndt, E.M., Lefebvre, A., Travis, F. and Munro, I.R., 1986, 'Fact and fantasy: psychosocial consequences of facial surgery in 24 Down syndrome children', *British Journal of Plastic Surgery,* 39, pp. 498-504,

Bailey, L.W., and Edwards, D, 1975, 'Psychological considerations in maxillo-facial prosthetics', *Journal of Prosthetic Dentistry,* 34,5, pp. 533-538.

Becker, H.S., (ed.) 1964, *The Other Side - Perspectives on Deviance,* New York: Free Press.

Bowlby, J., 1981, 'Loss: Sadness and Depression', *Attachment and Loss: Vol. III,* Harmondsworth: Penguin, p. 17.

Bull, R., and Stevens, J., 1981, 'The effects of facial disfigurement on helping behaviour', *The Italian Journal of Psychology,* Vol. viii, No. 1. April,

Bull, R., and Stevens, J., 1981, 'The relationship between ratings of persons' facial appearance and ratings of their conversations,' *Language and Speech,* Vol. 24, Part 3.

Bull, R., 1982, 'Physical Appearance and Criminality', *Current Psychological Reviews,* 2, pp. 269-282.

Bull, R., 1983, 'The General Public's Reaction to Facial Disfigurement', presented at the conference on *The Psychology of Cosmetic Treatment,* University of Pennsylvania, Philadelphia.

Constable, J.D., and Bernstein, N.R., 1979, 'Public and professional reactions to the facially disfigured which interfere with rehabilitation', *Scandinavian Journal of Plastic and Reconstructive Surgery*, 13, 1, pp. 181-183.

David, D.J., and Barritt, J.A., 1982 'Psychosocial implications of surgery for head and neck cancer', *Clinics in Plastic Surgery*, 9, 3, July.

Davis, F., 1961-2, 'Deviance Disavowal: the Management of Strained Interaction by the Visibly Handicapped', *Social Problems*, 9, pp. 120-132.

Erikson, K.T., 1962, 'Notes on the Sociology of Deviance', *The Other Side*, Becker, H.S., (ed.) a revision of a paper first published in Social Problems, Vol. 9 pp. 307-314.

Festinger, L., et al., 1964, *When Prophecy Fails*, Harper and Row, London.

Fiegenbaum, W., 1981, 'A social training program for clients with facial disfigurations: a contribution to the rehabilitation of cancer patients', *International Journal of Rehabilitation Research*, 4 (4), pp.501-509.

Frank, O.S., 1975, 'Psychosocial factors in the prosthetic rehabilitation of the facially disfigured patient', presented at the International Facial Prosthetic Workshop, Institute of Maxillo-facial Technology, pp. 142-145.

Friedenbergs, I., 1981, 'Psychosocial management of patients with cutaneous cancers', *Journal of Dermatologic Surgery and Oncology*, 7, 10, pp. 323-330.

Gaioni, K., 1988, 'Rx: Self-Help', *The New Physician*, July-August.

Goffman, E., 1955, 'On Face-Work: An Analysis of Ritual Elements Social Interaction', *Psychiatry*, Vol.18, No.3, pp.213-231, August, repeated in 1967, *Interaction Ritual: Essays on Face-to-Face Behaviour*, Doubleday Anchor, New York.

Goffman, E., 1956, 'Embarrassment and Social Interaction', *American Journal of Sociology*, Vol.62, No.23, November, pp. 264-271, printed in Goffman, E., 1967 *Interaction Ritual: Essays on Face-to-Face Behaviour*, Doubleday Anchor, New York.

Goffman, E., 1959, *The Presentation of Self in Everyday Life*, Doubleday Anchor, New York.

Goffman, E., 1961, *Asylums*, Anchor Books, New York, and 1968, Penguin, Harmondsworth.

Goffman, E., Stigma 1963, 'Notes on the Management of Spoiled Identity', Englewood Cliffs, Prentice-Hall, published 1968 Pelican, Harmondsworth.

Goffman, E., 1963, *Encounters: Two Studies in the Sociology of Interaction*, Bobbs-Merrill Co., Indianapolis.

Greenblatt, M. and Lindz, T., 1957, 'Some Dimensions of the Problem', *The Patient and the Mental Hospital*, Greenblatt, M., Levinson, D.J., and Williams, R.H., Glencoe, Free Press.

Homans, G.C., 1974, *Social Behaviour, Its Elementary Forms*, Harcourt Brace Jovanovich, New York.

Howell, M., and Ford, P., 1980, *The True History of the Elephant Man*, Allison and Busby, London.

Hunt, P.(ed.), 1966, *Stigma: the Experience of Disability*, Chapman, London.

Ildstad, S., Tollerud, D.J., Bigelow, M.E. and Remensnyder, J.P., 1989, 'A multivariate analysis of determinants of survival for patients with squamous cell carcinoma of the head and neck', *Ann. Surg.*, February, 209, 2, pp. 237-241.

Jackson, M., 1986, *The Boy David*, British Broadcasting Corporation, London.

Kalick, S.M., 1982, 'Clinician, Social Scientist and Body Image', *Clinics in Plastic Surgery* 9,3, pp.379-385, July,.

Lefebvre, A., and Munro, I.R., 1978, 'The role of psychiatry in a craniofacial team', *Plastic and Reconstructive Surgery*, April 61, 4, pp. 564-56.

Lefebvre, A., and Barclay, S., 1982, 'Psychosocial impact of craniofacial deformities before and after reconstructive surgery', *Canadian Journal of Psychiatry*, 27, 7, pp. 579-584.

Light, J., 1976, 'Psychological aspects of disability and rehabilitation of cancer patients', *New York Journal of Dentistry*, 46, 9, November, pp. 293-297.

Lofland, J., 1980, 'Early Goffman: Style, Structure, Substance, Soul', *The View from Goffman*, ed. Jason Ditton, Macmillan, London.

Macgregor, F.C., and Schaffner, B., 1950, 'Screening patients for nasal plastic operations', *Psychomatic Medicine*, 12, 5, pp. 277-291, September/October.

Macgregor, F.C., 1951, 'Some psycho-social problems associated with facial deformities', *American Sociological Review*, 16, 5, pp. 629-638, October.

Macgregor, F.C., 1953, 'Some psychological hazards of plastic surgery of the face', *Plastic and Reconstructive Surgery*, 12, 2,. Based on a lecture given at the American Academy of Ophthalmology and Otolaryngology, Chicago, 1951.

Macgregor, F.C., Abel, T.M., Bryt, A., Laner, E. and Weissmann, S., 1953, *Facial Deformities and Plastic Surgery: a Psychosocial Study*, Charles C. Thomas, Springfield, Ill.

Macgregor, F.C., 1967, 'Social and cultural components in the motivations of persons seeking plastic surgery of the nose', *Journal of Health and Social Behaviour*, 8, 2.

Macgregor, F.C., 1970, 'Social and psychological implications of dento-facial disfigurement', *The Angle Orthodontist*, 40, 3, pp. 231-233.

Macgregor, F.C., and Ford, B., 1971, 'The other face of plastic surgery: the disappointed patient', *Science Digest*, pp. 16-20, April.

Macgregor, F.C., 1973, 'Social and Psychological Considerations', chapter 3 of *Cosmetic Facial Surgery*, Rees, T.D. and Wood-Smith, D., Philadelphia: W.B. Saunders, p. 31.

Macgregor, F.C., 1973, 'Traumatic facial injuries and the law: some social, psychological and economic ramifications', *Trial Lawyers Quarterly*, Vol. 9, 4, Fall, pp. 50-53.

Macgregor, F.C., 1974, *Transformation and Identity - The Face and Plastic Surgery*, Quadrangle/The New York Times Book Company, New York.

Macgregor, F.C., 1976, 'Aesthetic plastic surgery: some caveats', *Aesthetic Plastic Surgery*, 1, 1 pp. 71-80.

Macgregor, F.C., 1978, 'Ear deformities: social and psychological implications', *Clinics in Plastic Surgery*, 5, 3, July.

Macgregor, F.C., 1979, *After Plastic Surgery (Adaptation and Adjustment)*, J.F. Bergin, New York.

Macgregor, F.C., 1980, 'The facially disfigured child', *Paediatric Social Work*, 1, 1.

Macgregor, F.C., 1981, 'Patient dissatisfaction with results of technically satisfactory surgery', *Aesthetic Plastic Surgery*, pp. 27-32.

Macgregor, F.C., 1982, 'Social and psychological studies of plastic surgery', *Clinics in Plastic Surgery*, 9, 3, pp. 283-288.

Macgregor, F.C., 1982, 'Surgery: the patient and the surgeon', *Clinics in Plastic Surgery*, 9, 3, pp. 387-395, July.

Macgregor, F.C., 1984, 'Psychic trauma of facial disfigurement', *Trial*, January.

Macgregor, F.C., 1984, 'Cosmetic surgery: a sociological analysis of litigation and a surgical speciality', *Aesthetic Plastic Surgery*, 8, pp. 219-224.

Mayo Foundation, 1988, 'Investment in the Future', *1987 Annual Report*, Mayo Foundation.

Morton, R.P., et al., 1984, 'Quality of life in treated head and neck cancer patients', *Clinical Otolaryngology*, 9, 3, pp. 81-185.

Munro, I.R., 1975, 'Orbito-cranio-facial surgery: the team approach', *Plastic and Reconstructive Surgery*, 55, 2, February, pp. 170-176.

Nordlicht, S., 1979, 'Facial disfigurement and psychiatric sequelae', *New York State Journal of Medicine*, 79, 9, pp. 1382-1384.

Page, R., 1984, *Stigma*, R.K.P., London.

Partridge, J., 1990, *Changing Faces - The Challenge of Facial Disfigurement*, Penguin, Harmondsworth.

Parkes, C.M., 1975, *Bereavement: Studies of Grief in Adult Life*, Penguin, Harmondsworth p.223.

Perlman, H.H., 1957, *Social Casework, a Problem-solving Process*, University of Chicago Press, Chicago, p. viii.

Peterson, L.J., and Topazian, R.G., 1974, 'The preoperative interview and psychological evaluation of the orthognathic surgery patient',*Journal of Oral Surgery*, 32, 8, pp. 583--588.

Piercy, M., 1978, *Woman on the Edge of Time*, Women's Press, London.

Piff, C., 1985, *Let's Face It*, Victor Gollancz, London.

Pinker, R., *The Idea of Welfare*, Heinemann, London.

Reid, W.J., and Epstein, L., 1972, *Task-Centred Casework*, Columbia Press, New York, p.21.

Reid, W.J., and Shyne, A., 1970, *Brief and Extended Casework*, Columbia Press, New York, p.vi.

Richmond, M., 1922, *What is Social Casework?* Russell Sage Foundation, New York.

Riley, C., 1968, 'Maxillo-facial prosthetic rehabilitation of postoperative cancer patients', *Journal of Prosthetic Dentistry*, October, 20, 4, pp. 352-360.

Roback, H.B., Kirshner, and Roback, E., 1981-2, 'Physical self-concept changes in a mildly facially disfigured neurofibromatosis patient following communication skill training', *International Journal of Psychiatry in Medicine*, 11, 2, pp. 137-143.

Roefs, A.J.M., van Oort, R.P., and Schaub, R.M.H., 1984, 'Factors related to the acceptance of facial prostheses', *The Journal of Prosthetic Dentistry*, Dec. 52, 6, pp. 849-852.

Rozen, R.D., Ordway, D.E., Curtis, T.A., and Cantor, R., 1972, 'Psychosocial aspects of maxillo-facial rehabilitation. Part 1. The effect of primary cancer treatment', *The Journal of Prosthetic Dentistry*, October, 28, 4, pp. 423-428.

Rumsey, N., Bull, R., and Gahagan, D., 1982, 'The effect of facial disfigurement on the proxemic behaviour of the general public', *Journal of Applied Social Psychology*, 12, 2, pp. 1397-150.

Rumsey, N., Bull, R., and Gahagan, D., 1986, 'A developmental study of children's stereotyping of facially deformed adults', *British Journal of Psychology*, 77, pp. 269-274.

Sainsbury, E., 1973, *Social Diagnosis in Casework*, Routledge and Kegan Paul, London, p.74.

Salmon, J., 1987 'Special People', *Let's Face It Newsletter*, April.

Schur, E., 1965, *Crimes Without Victims: deviant behaviour and public policy: abortion, homosexuality, drug addition*, Prentice-Hall, Englewood Cliffs, New Jersey.

Sela, M., and Lowental, U., 1980, 'Therapeutic effects of maxillo-facial prostheses', *Oral Surgery*, July, 50, 1, pp. 13-16.

Spicker, P., 1984, *Stigma and Social Welfare*, Croom Helm, Beckenham.

Stricker, G., et al., 1979, 'Psychosocial aspects of craniofacial disfigurement', *American Journal of Orthodontics*, 76, 4, pp. 410-422.

Szasz, T., 1971, *The Manufacture of Madness*, R.K.P., London.

Titmuss, R.M., 1973, *The Gift Relationship*, Penguin, Harmondsworth.

Trust, D.S., 1986, *Overcoming Disfigurement: defeating the problems - physical, social and emotional*, Thorsons, Wellingborough.

Van Doorne, J., 1981, 'Psychosocial aspects of cancer patients with facial disfigurement', *International Facial Prosthetic Workshop*, pp. 80-88.

Watson, D., 1980, *Caring for Strangers: an Introduction to Practical Philosophy for Students of Social Administration*, R.K.P., London, p. 57.

West, D.W., 1973, 'Adaptation to surgically induced facial disfigurement among cancer patients', referred to in 1974, *Dissertation Abstracts International*, 34, 7, p. 4442.

Weston, S., 1989, *Walking Tall*, Bloomsbury, London.

Wolfensberger, W., 1972, *The Principle of Normalisation in Human Services*, National Institute on Mental Retardation, Toronto.

Worden, J.W., 1983, *Grief Counselling and Grief Therapy*, Tavistock, London and New York, p. ix.

Printed and bound by CPI Group (UK) Ltd, Croydon, CR0 4YY

21/10/2024

01777086-0007